Y0-CRI-351

Ernst Schering Research Foundation Workshop 41
The Future of the Oocyte

Springer
Berlin
Heidelberg
New York
Hong Kong
London
Milan
Paris
Tokyo

Ernst Schering Research Foundation
Workshop 41

The Future of the Oocyte

Basic and Clinical Aspects

J. Eppig, Ch. Hegele-Hartung, M. Lessl
Editors

With 17 Figures

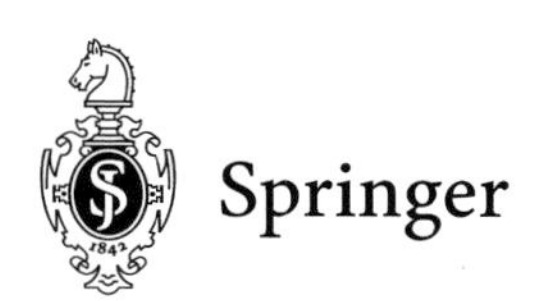

Springer

Series Editors: G. Stock and M. Lessl

ISSN 0947-6075
ISBN 3-540-43747-9 Springer-Verlag Berlin Heidelberg New York

Library of Congress Cataloging-in-Publication Data

The future of the oocyte : basic and clinical aspects / J. Eppig and Ch. Hegele-Hartung, editors.
p. cm. -- (Ernst Schering Research Foundation workshop, ISSN 0947-6075 ; 41)
Includes bibliographical references and index.
ISBN 3540437479 (alk. paper)
1. Ovum--Congresses. 2. Infertility, Female--Congresses. I. Eppig, J. (John) II. Hegele-Hartung, Ch. (Christa), 1954- III. Series.

Springer-Verlag Berlin Heidelberg New York
a member of BertelsmannSpringer Science+Business Media GmbH

http://www.springer.de

Typesetting: Data conversion by Springer-Verlag
Printing: Druckhaus Beltz, Hemsbach
Binding: J. Schäffer GmbH & Co. KG, Grünstadt
SPIN: 10865452 21/3130/AG–5 4 3 2 1 0 – Printed on acid-free paper

Preface

Although Reinier De Graaf (1641–1673) is considered the founder of modern reproductive biology, scientific knowledge of folliculo- and embryogenesis did not progress significantly until the nineteenth and (especially) twentieth centuries. The first successful transfer of an in vitro fertilized (IVF) human egg in 1976 by Steptoe and Edward was a milestone in modern reproductive biology. The first baby conceived through IVF was delivered in 1978. Since that time, modern endocrinology, genetics, and assisted reproductive technologies have opened new frontiers of research with the aim to treat infertile women. As a consequence, IVF is now a well-established treatment for female infertility, and new technologies based on oocyte biology hold the promise of even more startling clinical applications. Nevertheless, success rates using assisted reproductive technologies remain low, with only about 23% of women who undergo treatment becoming pregnant using IVF (HFES 2000). Efforts are being made to improve implantation rates after IVF by improving embryo culture conditions, optimizing oocyte quality, and developing new technologies of selecting viable embryos for transfer.

Besides increasing trends in assisted reproductive technologies, the major focus of clinical research is the manipulation of ovarian function by exogenous follicle-stimulating hormone (FSH) in an attempt to optimize follicular development. Improved understanding of mechanisms regulating early follicular development may give rise to more refined and individualized protocols to assist reproduction. For example, it is likely that ovarian stimulation protocols will eventually be replaced by the in vitro maturation of oocytes. However, our knowledge of follicu-

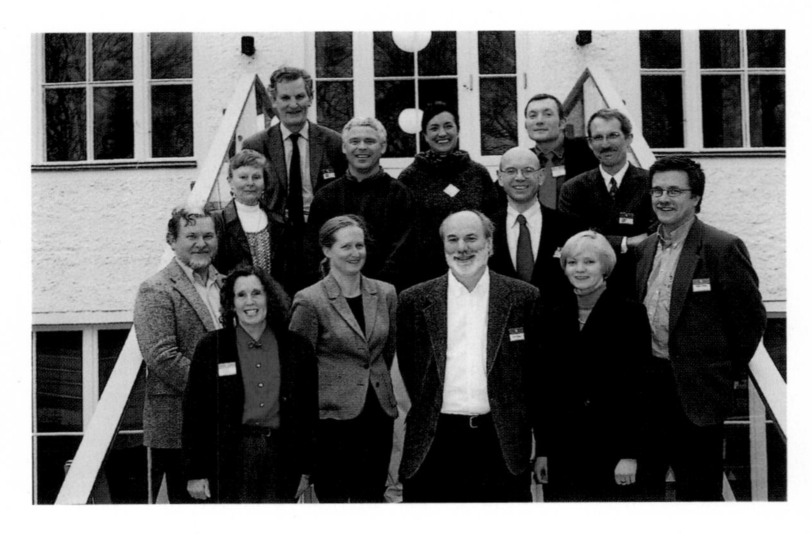

The participants of the workshop

logenesis and oocyte maturation is rudimentary, and the safety of in vitro maturation and other reproductive technologies remains to be established.

Current knowledge of many aspects of mammalian folliculogenesis, oocyte maturation, and fertilization is undergoing rapid advancement due to the application of knockout technologies using the mouse model (for example, *Zp3*$^{-/-}$ and *Gdf9*$^{-/-}$). Over the last 10 years, these transgenic mouse models have defined the roles of extraovarian and intraovarian factors in folliculogenesis and oocyte development. In this new century, more data will be generated in understanding ovarian and reproductive physiology using these mouse models and other genomic, pharmacogenomic, and proteomic approaches.

In this 2-day workshop, held January 2002 in Berlin, Germany, we set out to promote an interdisciplinary discussion – between experts from various fields of basic, company-based, and clinical research – related to folliculogenesis and oocyte development. The aim of this workshop was to present, discuss, and assess novel approaches in mammalian folliculogenesis and oocyte development that may have an impact on fertility/infertility in the near or distant future. Key issues were the understanding of new modulators of folliculogenesis and regulators of cytoplasmic as well as meiotic oocyte maturation, modern technologies, the aging oocyte, and pathogenic mechanisms of infertility. Areas covered in this workshop included studies concerning early and late follicular development and in vitro culture strategies of oocytes. Recent observations concerning the development of new compounds and regimens for ovarian stimulation were also discussed and were the basis for the outlook on therapeutic strategies that improve the balance between success and complications of assisted reproductive technologies.

We are indebted to the Ernst Schering Research Foundation for providing us with the necessary resources and help to organize this workshop. We wish to thank the authors for their contributions and the lively discussion at the workshop.

Berlin, April 2002
Christa Hegele-Hartung, John Eppig

Contents

1 Hormonal Control of Folliculogenesis: The Key to Successful Reproduction
D.T. Baird, A. Mitchell 1

2 Activation of Primordial Follicles
J.E. Fortune 11

3 Follicular Development and Apoptosis
H. Billig, E. Markström, E.C. Svensson, R. Shao, A. Friberg 23

4 Delivery of the Oocyte from the Follicle to the Oviduct: A Time of Vulnerability
J.S. Richards 43

5 Phenotypic Effects of Knockout of Oocyte-Specific Genes
S. Varani, M.M. Matzuk 63

6 The Biochemistry of Oocyte Maturation
S.M. Downs 81

7 The Structural Basis of Oocyte-Granulosa Cell Communication
D.F. Albertini 101

8 Ageing and Aneuploidy in Oocytes
U. Eichenlaub-Ritter 111

9 Ovarian Infertility – Reasons and Treatment Paradigms
M. Ludwig, K. Diedrich 137

10 Can Stimulation Protocols Improve Oocyte Quality?
J. Smitz 161

11 FF-MAS and Its Role in Mammalian Oocyte Maturation
C. Grøndahl 177

Subject Index 195

Previous Volumes Published in This Series 197

List of Editors and Contributors

Editors

Eppig, J.
The Jackson Laboratory, 600 Main Street, Bar Harbor, ME 04609, USA
e-mail: Jje@aretha.jax.org

Hegele-Hartung, Ch.
Safety Pharm. Mgmt., Schering AG, Müllerstr. 178, 13342 Berlin, Germany
e-mail: christa.hegelehartung@schering.de

Lessl, M.
Female Health Care, Schering AG, Müllerstr. 178, 13342 Berlin, Germany
e-mail: monika.lessl@schering.de

Contributors

Albertini, D.F.
Department and Cellular Biology, Tuft University School of Medicine,
136 Harrison Avenue, Boston, MA 02111, USA
e-mail: David.albertini@tufts.edu

Baird, D.T.
Department of Obstetrics and Gynecology, Centre for Reproductive Biology,
University of Edinburgh, 37 Chalmers Street, Edinburgh, EH3 9ET, UK
e-mail: dtbaird@ed.ac.uk

Billig, H.
Department of Physiology, Göteborg University, P.O. Box 434,
40530 Göteborg, Sweden
e-mail: hakan.billig@fysiologi.gu.se

Diedrich, K.
Department of Gynecology and Obstetrics Medical University of Lübeck,
Ratzeburger Allee 160, 23538 Lübeck, Germany
e-mail: Diedrich@medinf.mu-luebeck.de

Downs, S.M.
Biology Department, Marquette University, 503 N 15 St.
Milwaukee, WI 53233, USA
e-mail: Downss@marquette.edu

Eichenlaub-Ritter, U.
Faculty of Biology, University of Bielefeld, Universitätsstr. 26,
33615 Bielefeld, Germany
e-mail: EiRi@biologie.uni-bielefeld.de

Fortune, J.E.
Cornell University, Department of Biomedical Sciences, Ithaca, NY 14853,
USA
e-mail: JF11@cornell.edu

Friberg, A.
Department of Physiology, Göteborg University, P.O. Box 434,
40530 Göteborg, Sweden
e-mail: chgr@novonordisk.com

Grøndahl, C.
Novo Nordisk A/S, Health Care, Health Care Fertility Team, Sauntesvej 13,
2820 Gentofte, Denmark
e-mail: chgr@novonordisk.com

Ludwig, M.
Department of Gynecology and Obstetrics, Medical University of Lübeck
Ratzeburger Allee 160, 23538 Lübeck, Germany
e-mail: Ludwig_M@t-online.de

Markström, E.
Department of Physiology, Göteborg University, P.O. Box 434,
40530 Göteborg, Sweden
e-mail: emilia.markstrom@fysiologi.gu.se

Matzuk, M.M.
Departments of Pathology, Baylor College of Medicine,
Molecular and Cellular Biology and Molecular and Human Genetics,
Room S217, One Baylor Plaza, Houston, TX 77030, USA
e-mail: Mmatzuk@bcm.tmc.edu

Mitchell, A.
Department of Obstetrics and Gynecology, Centre for Reproductive Biology,
University of Edinburgh, 37 Chalmers Street, Edinburgh, EH3 9ET, UK
e-mail: amitchell@ed-ac.uk

Richards, J.S.
Department of Molecular and Cellular Biology, Baylor College of Medicine,
One Baylor Plaza, Houston, TX 77030, USA
e-mail: Joanner@bcm.tmc.edu

Shao, R.
Department of Physiology, Göteborg University, P.O. Box 434,
40530 Göteborg, Sweden
e-mail: ruijin.shao@fysiologi.gu.se

Smitz, J.
Follicle Biology Laboratory, Vrije Universiteit Brussel, Laarbeklaan 101,
1090 Brussels, Belgium
e-mail: Johan.Smitz@az.vub.ac.be

Svensson, E.C.
Department of Physiology, Göteborg University, P.O. Box 434,
40530 Göteborg, Sweden
e-mail: eva.svensson@fysiologi.gu.se

Varani, S.
Baylor College of Medicine, Department of Pathology, One Baylor Plaza,
Houston, TX 77030, USA
e-mail: svarani@bcm.tmc.edu

1 Hormonal Control of Folliculogenesis: The Key to Successful Reproduction

D.T. Baird, A. Mitchell

1.1 Introduction 1
1.2 Primary Recruitment 2
1.3 Development of Preantral Follicles 3
1.4 Antral Follicle Development 4
1.5 Secondary Recruitment and Selection of the Dominant Follicle(s) . . 4
References 7

1.1 Introduction

Folliculogenesis is the process by which primordial follicles are promoted through a series of developmental steps until a mature oocyte is ovulated. The process of folliculogenesis is not fully understood and involves initial or primary recruitment from the primordial pool, development of small primary and secondary preantral follicles, formation of an antral cavity, and finally the selection of the ovulatory follicle(s) (Hirshfield 1991; Gougeon 1996). The growth and differentiation of the oocyte and the surrounding somatic cells which make up the follicle are subject to various carefully regulated steps which ensure that the number of eggs which are ovulated is reduced to that which is appropriate for the species. The disastrous consequences of dysregulation of this system are illustrated by sheep carrying the Booroola fecundity gene (Baird and Campbell 1998). Due to a mutation in the $BMPRI_{\beta}$ receptor, these sheep ovulate up to ten eggs instead of one or two (de Souza et al.

2001; Mulsant et al. 2001; Wilson et al. 2001). The subsequent fetuses die due to either abortion or following premature birth. As a result, under natural circumstances the mutation only rarely persists in those few ewes carrying a single copy of the gene which ovulates twins.

In this paper I shall review the hormonal control of the key steps in folliculogenesis with particular reference to man. Much of the evidence concerning the early stages of recruitment and follicle development is derived from research in experimental animals, particularly rodents, and will be discussed later in the symposium. Although the time scale of follicle development ranges from approximately 1 month in rats and mice to nearly 6 months in women and sheep, the basic molecular mechanisms are likely to be similar. Indeed, the process involving extensive changes in morphology and function is analogous to morphogenesis during embryonic and fetal development. It is not surprising, therefore, that many of the same genes are expressed, e.g., transforming growth factor (TGF)-β family of growth factors.

1.2 Primary Recruitment

Primitive germ cells (PGS) migrate from the dorsal endoderm of the yolk sac during fetal life to the genital ridge where they divide and differentiate into oogonia (Mauleon 1978). The surrounding somatic cells which form the granulosa and theca cells associate with the oocyte to form the pool of primordial follicles from which follicles will be recruited throughout reproductive life. Meiosis is arrested at the dictyate stage of the first meiotic division in these resting oocytes and does not recommence until a few hours before ovulation. Every day a small fraction of the pool is recruited for further development (primary recruitment). The factors which determine the rate of primary recruitment are not fully understood. It is unlikely that blood-borne classical hormones are involved because recruitment continues before puberty, during pregnancy and lactation at the same rate although the levels of gonadotrophins and steroids are markedly different (Gougeon 1996). As the total number of oocytes in the ovaries declines with age, a greater proportion of the residual pool is recruited, although the absolute number is reduced (Krarup et al. 1969). If the total number is reduced experimentally by hemicastration or irradiation, there is a compensatory increase in the proportion of primordial follicles without any significant long-term change in the levels of gonadotrophins.

The most plausible explanation for the increased recruitment is a reduction in some inhibitory factor produced by adjacent developing follicles. Recent evidence in support of this hypothesis has been provided from experiments where strips of ovarian cortex from sheep and cattle containing antral follicles were cultured in vitro (Wandji et al. 1996). In the absence of adjacent developing follicles, there was massive recruitment of primordial follicles into the growing phase. In experiments when the strips were autotransplanted in vivo, the increased rate of recruitment was maintained until the development of antral follicles at 120 days (D.T. Baird, B.K. Campbell, C.J.H. de Souza, and E. Telfer, unpublished data). The nature of the factor or factors influencing recruitment is not known, although anti-Müllerian hormone (AMH) inhibits recruitment in neonatal mouse ovaries (Durlinger et al. 1999).

1.3 Development of Preantral Follicles

As recruitment of primordial follicles and development of preantral follicles continues following hypophysectomy, traditionally it has been considered that gonadotrophins are not involved in the early stages of follicle development (Gougeon 1996). However, mRNA for follicle-stimulating hormone (FSH) receptor has been detected by RT-PCR on the granulosa cells of some primary and secondary follicles in women (O'Shaughnessy et al. 1996; Oktay et al. 1997). Whether functional receptors are present is not known, but there is evidence that the rate of preantral development is sensitive to gonadotrophins. Hypophysectomy of fetal monkeys (Gulyas et al. 1977) or treatment of neonatal rats with gonadotrophin-releasing hormone (GnRH) antagonist (McGee et al. 1997) reduces the number of developing follicles and increases the rate of atresia. In addition, treatment with FSH enhances the rate of development of primordial follicles. Thus, although development of primordial follicles *can* occur in the absence of gonadotrophins, it is likely that follicles become increasingly responsive to FSH even before an antrum is formed.

It is likely that preantral follicles are influenced by a range of other local paracrine factors at different stages of development. Many of these "survival" factors interact with FSH and luteinizing hormone (LH) even in preantral follicles to modify the action of gonadotrophins. For example, in many in vitro systems activin enhances the ability of FSH to induce aromatase in granulosa cells (Miro et al. 1991; Xiao et al. 1992). In contrast, activin A inhibits the ability of FSH to stimulate the growth of small primary follicles in adult mice (Yokota et al. 1997). Moreover, coculture with larger secondary follicles inhibits the growth of primary follicles, an effect which can be neutralized by the addition of follistatin (Mizunuma et al. 1999). These experiments illustrate that local factors arising from adjacent follicles at different stages of development can interact with gonadotrophins and other systemic factors to influence the growth and development of the preantral follicles.

1.4 Antral Follicle Development

Once an antrum is formed the follicle becomes dependent on gonadotrophins. FSH is necessary for the formation of the antrum, which occurs in humans when the follicle reaches approximately 0.1 mm. From this point onwards, the follicle becomes increasingly sensitive to the fluctuations in the levels of gonadotrophins in blood. A certain minimal level of FSH is required to sustain full growth; atresia ensues if the level falls below this threshold level (Baird 1983).

1.5 Secondary Recruitment and Selection of the Dominant Follicle(s)

In the few days prior to ovulation, the number of healthy large antral follicles is reduced to the number appropriate for that species. In monovular species like cow and human, only a single ovulatory follicle emerges, while the remainder undergo atresia. The process by which a single follicle is selected for ovulation from the cohort of small antral follicles of a similar stage of development is not fully understood. It involves three crucial steps: (1) secondary recruitment, (2) selection, and (3) dominance.

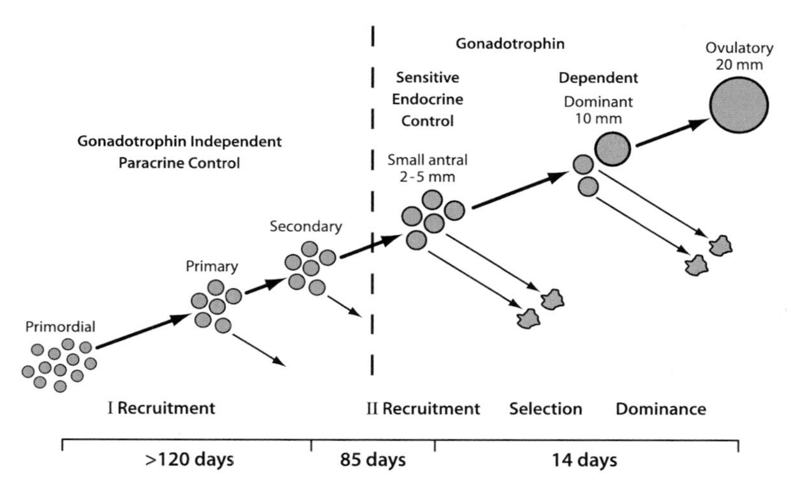

Fig. 1. Folliculogenesis in women. The *dashed line* indicates the time of antrum formation (0.1–0.2 mm diameter)

1.5.1 Secondary Recruitment

Secondary recruitment occurs from the pool of healthy small antral follicles (2–4 mm diameter) which are present in the ovary at the time of luteal regression. As the levels of estradiol, progesterone, and inhibin A fall, the secretion of FSH and LH increases. The concentration of FSH rises above that required to activate the mechanisms necessary for the final differentiation of the follicles, including stimulation of aromatase and LH receptors in the granulosa cells. This maturational process is reflected by a rise in the peripheral concentration of inhibin B, which occurs within 48 h of the rise in FSH (Groome et al. 1996). mRNA for activin/inhibin β_B subunit is present in granulosa cells of even preantral follicles (McNatty et al. 2000). In contrast, inhibin α-subunit expression occurs only around the time of antrum formation (Fig. 1). Following injection of FSH in women, there is an immediate rise in the concentration of both inhibin A and B (Anderson et al. 1998). It is likely, therefore, that the rise in inhibin B concentration observed during the luteal to follicular transition represents stimulation of the cohort of small antral follicles by FSH.

1.5.2 Selection

How is a single follicle "selected" from this cohort? The most plausible hypothesis is based on the presumption that all the follicles in the cohort are not at exactly the same stage of development. Although of similar size, one follicle is presumed to be slightly more developed so it can respond immediately to the intercycle rise in FSH. A number of intraovarian factors are known to alter the responsiveness of the granulosa and theca cells to FSH and LH. For example, activin and insulin-like growth factor (IGF)I and/or II enhance the ability of FSH to induce aromatase (Campbell 1999). Thus the "chosen" follicle is able to benefit maximally from the intercycle rise in FSH and develop at a faster rate than other subordinate follicles.

1.5.3 Dominance

Once selected, it is essential that the dominant follicle suppresses the further development of other antral follicles which have the potential to ovulate. The mechanism involves suppression of FSH below the threshold necessary to activate and sustain the growth and development of other follicles. The marked rise in the concentration of inhibin A and estradiol in the mid- and late-follicular phase of the cycle is derived almost exclusively from the dominant follicle (Groome et al. 1996). In this way, the ovulatory follicle has total control over the feedback signals which control the secretion of gonadotrophins by the anterior pituitary.

How does the dominant follicle maintain the final stages of growth and development in the face of declining levels of FSH? There are at least two likely mechanisms. Around the time of selection, the granulosa cells of the dominant follicle acquire significant numbers of LH receptors (Webb and England 1982). In the follicular phase of the cycle the levels of LH, in contrast to those of FSH, rise in association with a marked increase in the frequency of LH pulses (Baird 1978). This rise in LH stimulates increased production of androgen from the theca, which ensures an abundant supply of precursor for estradiol synthesis. In addition, as the granulosa cells acquire LH receptors, they can increasingly utilize LH as well as FSH via the generation of cyclic adenosine monophosphate (cAMP). In this way the late follicular phase LH may be used as a partial surrogate for FSH to promote the final stage of folliculogenesis.

It is likely that local autocrine and paracrine factors also increase the sensitivity of the dominant follicle to FSH. As mentioned above, IGF enhances the responsiveness of granulosa cells to FSH in vitro. In small follicles the bulk of IGF is inactivated by binding to IGFBP. In some species there is a high concentration of unbound IGF in the preovulatory follicle due to the selective degradation of IGFBP (Mazerbourg et al. 2000; Fortune et al. 2001). It is likely that inhibin and estradiol act locally within the follicle, as well as acting as key endocrine signals. In several species it has been demonstrated that inhibin enhances LH stimulated androgen production by theca (Hillier et al. 1991), and FSH stimulated aromatase activity in sheep granulosa cells (Campbell and Baird 2001). In this way the dominant follicle becomes increasingly sensitive to gonadotrophins and can survive in an environment which is hostile to the recruitment and further development of subordinate follicles.

References

Anderson RA, Groome NP, Baird DT (1998) Inhibin A and inhibin B in women with polycystic ovarian syndrome during treatment with FSH to induce mono-ovulation. Clin Endocrinol (Oxf) 48:577–584

Baird DT (1978) Pulsatile secretion of LH and ovarian estradiol during the follicular phase of the sheep estrous cycle. Biol Reprod 18:359–364

Baird DT (1983) Factors regulating the growth of preovulatory follicle in the sheep and human. J Reprod Fertil 69:343–352

Baird DT, Campbell BK (1998) Follicle selection in sheep with breed differences in ovulation rate. Mol Cell Endocrinol 145:89–95

Campbell BK (1999) The modulation of gonadotrophic hormone action on the ovary by paracrine and autocrine factors. Anat Histol Embryol 28:247–251

Campbell BK, Baird DT (2001) Inhibin A is a follicle stimulating hormone-responsive marker of granulosa cell differentiation, which has both autocrine and paracrine actions in sheep. J Endocrinol 169:333–345

de Souza CJH, MacDougall C, Campbell BK, et al (2001) The Booroola (FecB) phenotype is associated with a mutation in the bone morphogenic receptor type IB (BMPRIB) gene. J Endocrinol 169:R1–R6

Durlinger AL, Kramer P, Karels B, et al (1999) Control of primordial follicle recruitment by anti-Müllerian hormone in the mouse ovary. Endocrinol 140:5789–5796

Fortune JE, Rivera GM, et al (2001) Differentiation of dominant versus subordinate follicles in cattle. Biol Reprod 65:648–654

Gougeon A (1996) Regulation of ovarian follicular development in primates: facts and hypotheses. Endocr Rev 17:121–155

Groome NP, Illingworth PJ, O'Brien M, et al (1996) Measurement if dimeric inhibin B throughout the human menstrual cycle. J Clin Endocrinol Metab 81:1401–1405

Gulyas BJ, Hodgen GD, Tullner WW, et al (1977) Effects of fetal or maternal hypophysectomy on endocrine organs and body weight in infant rhesus monkeys (Macaca mulatta): with particular emphasis on oogenesis. Biol Reprod 16:216–227

Hillier SG, Yong EL, Illingworth PJ, et al (1991) Effects of recombinant inhibin on androgen synthesis in cultured human thecal cells. Mol Cell Endocrinol 75:R1–R6

Hirshfield AN (1991) Development of follicles in the mammalian ovary. Int Rev Cytol 124:43–101

Krarup T, Pederson T, Faber M, (1969) Regulation of oocyte growth in the mouse ovary. Nature 224:187–188

Mauleon P (1978) Ovarian development in young mammals. In: Crighton DB, Foxcroft GR, Lamming GE (eds) Control of ovulation. Butterworths, London, pp 141–158

Mazerbourg S, Zapf J, Bar RS, et al (2000) Insulin-like growth factor (IGF) –binding protein-4 proteolytic degradation in bovine, equine and porcine preovulatory follicles: regulation by IGFs and heparin-binding domain-containing peptides. Biol Reprod 63:390–400

McGee EA, Perlas E, LaBolt EA, et al (1997) Follicle-stimulating hormone enhances the development of preantral follicles in juvenile rats. Biol Reprod 57:990–998

McNatty KP, Fidler AE, Juengel JL, et al (2000) Growth and paracrine factors regulating follicular formation and cellular function. Mol Cell Endocrinol 163:11–20

Miro F, Smyth CD, et al (1991) Development-related effects of recombinant activin on steroid synthesis in rat granulosa cells. Endocrinol 129:3388–3394

Mizunuma H, Liu X, Andoh K, et al (1999) Activin from secondary follicles causes small preantral follicles to remain dormant at the resting stage. Endocrinol 140:37–42

Mulsant P, Lecerf F, Fabrie S, et al (2001) Mutation in bone morphogenetic protein receptor-IB is associated with increased ovulation rate in Booroola Merino ewes. Proc Natl Acad Sci USA 98:5104–5109

Oktay K, Briggs D, Gosden RG (1997) Ontogeny of follicle-stimulating hormone receptor gene expression in isolated human ovarian follicles. J Clin Endocrinol Metab 82:3748–3751

O'Shaughnessy PJ, Dudley K, Rajapaksha WR (1996) Expression of follicle stimulating hormone-receptor mRNA during gonadal development. Mol Cell Endocrinol 125:169–175

Wandji SA, Srsen V, Voss AF, et al (1996) Initiation in vitro of growth of bovine primordial follicles. Biol Reprod 55:942–948

Webb R, England G (1982) Identification of the ovulatory follicle in the ewe: associated changes in follicular size, thecal and granulosa cell luteinizing hormone receptors, antral fluid steroid, and circulating hormones during the preovulatory period. Endocrinol 110:873–881

Wilson T, Wu X-Y, Juengel JL, et al (2001) Highly prolific Booroola sheep have a mutation in the intracellular kinase domain of bone morphogenic protein IB receptor (ALK-6) that is expressed both in oocytes and granulosa cells. Biol Reprod 64:1225–1235

Xiao S, Robertson DM, Findlay JK (1992) Effects of activin and follicle-stimulating hormone (FSH) –suppressing protein/follistatin on FSH receptors and differentiation of cultured rat granulosa cells. Endocrinol 131:1009–1016

Yokota H, Yamada K, Liu X (1997) Paradoxical action of activin A on folliculogenesis in immature and adult mice. Endocrinol 138:4572–4576

2 Activation of Primordial Follicles

J.E. Fortune

2.1 Introduction 11
2.2 Overview of Species and Approaches Used to Study Activation of Primordial Follicles 12
2.3 Organ Cultures of Cortical Pieces from Ovaries of Cattle and Baboons (In Vitro) 14
2.4 CAM Grafts of Bovine Ovarian Cortical Pieces and Whole Mouse Ovaries (In Ovo) 15
2.5 Growth of Activated Follicles 17
2.6 Summary and Conclusions 18
References 19

2.1 Introduction

The development of ovarian follicles is a protracted process. Even in rodents, it is estimated to take about 8 weeks for development from the primordial to the preovulatory stage (Hirshfield 1991), and estimates for larger mammals like humans and cattle are around 6 months (Gougeon 1996). Although follicular growth and differentiation are gradual and continuous processes, there are critical transitional points in follicular development. They include initiation of follicular growth, selection of a dominant follicle capable of ovulating, and the transformation of a preovulatory follicle into a periovulatory follicle in response to the luteinizing hormone/follicle-stimulating hormone (LH/FSH) surge. This review will focus on the first of these critical transitions, the initiation of follicular growth. Understanding the signals that regulate the activation of primordial follicles is of practical importance since it could stimulate new ideas for contraceptive approaches or lead to methods to enhance fertility in women, domestic animals, and endangered species.

In mammals, ovarian follicles are first formed during fetal life (primates and ruminants) or around the time of birth (rodents). As soon as follicle formation has occurred, some of the newly formed follicles leave the resting pool and begin to grow. This process is referred to as "follicle activation" or "initiation of follicle growth." Although some progress has been made in identifying factors that may regulate follicle activation, the process is still very poorly understood. Even less well understood is what regulates the timing of follicle activation. Why do some follicles initiate growth soon after they are formed whereas others remain quiescent for months, years, or even decades, depending on the species? This review will provide a short overview of the species and general approaches that have been used to investigate the tantalizing mystery of follicular activation and a more in-depth review of the experimental models that my laboratory has developed for studying this critical transition and a summary of the findings they have generated.

2.2 Overview of Species and Approaches Used to Study Activation of Primordial Follicles

Rodents offer a number of advantages for studying the initiation of follicle growth. Follicle formation, in which an oocyte in the dictyate phase of prophase I becomes surrounded by a layer of flattened granulosa cells, occurs on the day of birth or shortly thereafter, depending on the species and strain of rodent. A subset of these follicles begins to grow just after their formation (Hirshfield 1991). The synchronicity of follicle formation and of the initiation of follicle growth, coupled with the small size of the newborn rodent ovary, offer unique experimental advantages. Intact ovaries can be cultured with putative regulators of follicular growth initiation and analyzed by histological or biochemical methods before and at various points during culture. In contrast, larger mammals offer none of these advantages, since follicle formation and the initiation of follicle growth occur during fetal life, usually during the last third of gestation (Henricson and Rajakowski 1959; van Wagenen and Simpson 1965; Russe 1983). In addition, these processes are not synchronous; follicle formation spans several weeks and some follicles initiate growth while others are still being formed. The ovaries, even the fetal ovary, are too large to be cultured as an intact unit. Nonetheless, these larger mammals, especially humans and domestic animals, are the species of practical interest. Hence, it is important to develop methods for studying the regulation of follicular development in primates and domestic animals. Since primordial follicles reside in the outer portion of the ovary, the ovarian cortex, my laboratory developed two experimental models that utilize small pieces of ovarian cortex, isolated from the rest of the ovary. Those methods will be discussed at greater length below.

Several different approaches have been taken to the question of what regulates follicle activation. One method is to simply examine follicles at various stages of early development for the expression of molecules (e.g., growth factors, receptors) of interest or their messenger RNAs (mRNAs), using in situ hybridization or immunohistochemistry. Results obtained with this approach have been reviewed recently by Picton (2001) and McNatty et al. (2000). In contrast to this descriptive approach, some investigators have cultured newborn mouse or rat ovaries with compounds hypothesized to be involved in follicle activation and then examined the ovaries histologically for evidence of effects on follicular dynamics. Studies using this type of approach have implicated various growth factors (reviewed by Nilsson and Skinner 2001), nerve growth factor and other neurotropins (Dissen et al. 2001), and anti-Müllerian hormone (Durlinger et al. 2002) as regulators of follicle activation. As mentioned above, somewhat different methods have been developed for studying initiation of follicle growth in ovaries of larger mammals. My laboratory (Wandji et al. 1996, 1997) and that of Braw-Tal (Braw-Tal and Yossefi 1997) independently developed a method in which small pieces of bovine ovarian cortex are organ-cultured. More recently, we developed a method for growing pieces of bovine or baboon ovarian cortex beneath the chorioallantoic membrane of chick embryos (Cushman et al. 2002). Results derived from these experimental approaches will be described in more detail below.

2.3 Organ Cultures of Cortical Pieces from Ovaries of Cattle and Baboons (In Vitro)

Pieces of ovarian cortex obtained from fetal ovaries of ruminants and primates during the last third of gestation contain large numbers of primordial follicles and a much smaller number of primary follicles. When cortical pieces from fetal bovine or baboon ovaries were placed in organ culture in Waymouth's medium supplemented with ITS+ (insulin, transferrin, selenium+linoleic acid and BSA), most follicles activated by day 2 of culture (Wandji et al. 1996, 1997). Granulosa cells had assumed the cuboidal shape typical of the primary follicle and follicle and oocyte diameter gradually increased with time in culture (10–20 days). Another series of experiments was conducted to define more closely the time of activation in vitro and the results showed that the majority of follicles left the resting pool between 12 and 24 h of culture (Fortune et al. 2000). This wholesale spontaneous activation of primordial follicles was unexpected and does not appear to be due to the fetal source of the material, since Braw-Tal and Yossefi (1997) reported that most follicles in cortical pieces from adult bovine ovaries also initiated growth spontaneously. In addition, proliferating cell nuclear antigen (PCNA), a marker for cell growth and proliferation, was expressed intensely in the follicles activated in vitro but absent in primordial follicles (Wandji et al. 1996, 1997).

The results suggest that follicle activation in vivo is regulated, at least in part, by an inhibitor(s) emanating from the inner, medullary region of the ovary. This hypothesis derives support from the finding that in cultures of whole, newborn mouse ovaries follicular development after 8 days in vitro was qualitatively similar to age-matched in vivo controls (Eppig and O'Brien 1996). However, attempts to restrain follicle activation in bovine cortical pieces by co-culture with pieces of medulla, or by leaving a piece of medulla attached to the cortex, have not supported that hypothesis, since the inclusion of medulla had no effect on the degree of follicle activation (Derrar et al. 2000; Fortune et al. 2000). However, if the medulla produces a diffusible inhibitory factor, its concentration may be too low in a co-culture situation in which the factor would be diluted by diffusion into the medium. Results from experiments with whole, newborn mouse ovaries discussed below lend support to the notion that the ovary may produce a diffusible inhibitory factor that becomes diluted in vitro. An alternative hypothesis is that the environment in vitro is actually richer in nutrients, growth factors, and/or hormones than the poorly vascularized (van Wezel and Rodgers 1996; Herrmann and Spanel-Borowski 1998) ovarian cortex in vivo and that this enriched environment triggers the mass exodus from the resting follicle pool.

2.4 CAM Grafts of Bovine Ovarian Cortical Pieces and Whole Mouse Ovaries (In Ovo)

The experiments summarized above showed that almost all follicles in cortical pieces from bovine and baboon ovaries initiate follicular growth in vitro in the absence of serum or specific growth factors or hormones. Although follicles readily and spontaneously developed to the primary stage, few follicles developed to the secondary stage, even when fetal calf serum was added to the medium (Fortune et al. 1999). We hypothesized that grafting bovine or baboon cortical pieces to the chorioallantoic membrane (CAM) of chick embryos would allow their vascularization and hence might hasten the development of newly activated follicles. Grafting tissues or organs to the surface of the chick CAM is a classical technique of embryology (Rudnick 1944; Rawles 1952). Such transplants are usually vascularized readily and can be observed or treated experimentally to improve understanding of developmental processes. Initial experiments, in which pieces of bovine ovarian cortex were placed on the outer surface of the CAM (the "traditional" position) were not successful at eliciting vascularization. Therefore, we developed a modified method that consists of placing a piece of bovine or baboon ovarian cortex beneath the CAM (between the CAM and the yolk sac membrane) on day 6 post-fertilization (Cushman et al. 2002). The grafts became vascularized rapidly. To our surprise, the wholesale, spontaneous activation observed in cortical pieces in vitro was completely absent "in ovo." The number of primordial and primary follicles was not significantly different after 10 days in ovo compared with day 0. In addition, this apparent inhibition of activation was reversible since pieces transferred to organ culture after 2 days beneath the CAM exhibited the usual activation of the majority of primordial follicles (Cushman et al. 2002). The reciprocal transfer, from in vitro to in ovo, was not as successful. The activated follicles present after 2 days in vitro gradually became atretic in ovo. It is possible that the shock of transfer and/or delay in the establishment of a blood supply is more detrimental to these growing follicles than to the non-growing primordial follicles in freshly isolated cortical pieces.

Although these results were radically different from what we had hypothesized, they are very intriguing and suggest the hypothesis that chick embryos have a specific inhibitor of follicle activation. We hypothesized that if there is such an inhibitor, its effects should be exerted on primordial follicles in whole ovaries, as well as those in ovarian cortical pieces. To test this hypothesis the ovaries of newborn C57BL/6J mice were grafted beneath the CAM of 6-day-old chick embryos and retrieved and fixed for histological morphometry after 8 days (Cushman et al. 2001). Controls included ovaries fixed: (1) on the day of birth, (2) after 8 days in vivo, and (3) after 8 days in vitro. Morphometric analysis of these four groups showed that, as expected (Eppig and O'Brien 1996), ovaries had only primordial follicles on the day of birth, but had developed primary and secondary follicles by day 8 in vivo or in vitro. Interestingly, there were significantly more growing (primary+secondary) follicles after 8 days in vitro vs in vivo; both the absolute number and percentage of growing follicles were greater in vitro. Although Eppig and O'Brien (1996) showed previously that the distribution of follicles among developmental classes is qualitatively similar after 8 days in vivo and in vitro, our results show that there are quantitative differences. These differences suggest that the rate of follicle activation is faster in vitro than in vivo. This could be due to the diffusion of an ovarian inhibitor of activation into the culture medium, resulting in lower concentrations of the inhibitor within the tissue in vitro vs in vivo. Whole mouse ovaries grafted beneath the CAM became vascularized, and in striking contrast to the day-8 in vitro and in vivo groups, only a very small number and percentage of growing follicles were present. These results are similar to those for CAM grafts of bovine and baboon cortical pieces and support the hypothesis that chick embryos produce a powerful inhibitor of follicle activation.

If there is such an inhibitor, it may be anti-Müllerian hormone (AMH). In mutant mice devoid of AMH, the follicular pool was depleted earlier in life compared with wildtype; heterozygotes exhibited an intermediate phenotype (Durlinger et al. 1999). In addition, AMH inhibits follicle activation in cultured newborn mouse ovaries (Durlinger et al. 2002). Since chick gonads of both sexes produce AMH (DiClemente et al. 1992), it may be the inhibitor in ovo. Although further experiments are needed to test this hypothesis, our preliminary studies showed that destruction of the embryonic chick gonads allows activation of primordial follicles in CAM grafts of bovine ovarian cortex (R.A. Cushman, C.M. Wahl and J.E. Fortune, unpublished data).

The culture of bovine and baboon cortical pieces in ovo provides a complementary experimental system to culture in vitro. Since almost all follicles activate in vitro, this may provide a good system for testing putative inhibitors of follicle growth initiation. The complete lack of activation in ovo provides an experimental system for testing potential stimulators of activation, as well as for determining the nature of the endogenous chick inhibitor.

2.5 Growth of Activated Follicles

The pool of resting primordial follicles is a tremendous potential resource for alleviation of infertility or for increasing the propagation of valuable domestic animals or endangered species, as well as a potential target for new contraceptives. However, successful use of the pool to increase fertility depends not only on the ability to activate primordial follicles in vitro, but also on the ability to successfully grow the activated follicles in vitro to the stage of meiotic and developmental competence of the oocyte. Although one live mouse has been produced from a follicle activated and grown in vitro, the course of both follicular and oocyte development is more protracted in mammals with larger follicles, such as primates and domestic animals. Thus, it may be even more difficult to achieve complete follicular development in vitro in these species than in rodents. Numerous studies have focused on growing bovine follicles from the medium-sized preantral stage to the antral stage, but growth from the primordial stage to the medium-sized preantral stage in vitro appears to be more difficult to achieve.

The organ culture system that we developed for activating primordial follicles may provide a good system for studying the next stage of follicular development, from the primary follicle to the preantral follicle with multiple layers of granulosa cells. It is difficult to estimate how long this stage of development normally takes in vivo, but estimates are as high as several months (Gougeon 1996). However, it is quite possible that normal development could be achieved in vitro more quickly. Therefore, we have tried to find culture conditions that would maximize growth and development of follicles in organ cultures of ovarian cortical pieces. Various doses of FSH and activin, both alone and in combination, had no effect on follicular dynamics in vitro (Fortune et al. 1998, 2000). Although an increase in cyclic AMP could be induced by adding forskolin or vasoactive intestinal peptide (VIP), FSH did not cause any change in cyclic AMP production even when forskolin or VIP, which both induce FSH responsiveness in follicles of newborn rats (Mayerhofer et al. 1997), was added for 8 h before treatment with FSH (Fortune et al. 1999). When cortical pieces were cultured with various concentrations of fetal bovine serum (FBS) with or without ITS+, the most effective treatments for the development of two-layered secondary follicles were 5% or 10% FBS in combination with 0.5×ITS+; these were much more effective than any concentration of FBS alone. The concentration of insulin in ITS+ is high enough (6.25 μg/ml) to suggest that insulin might be acting through the insulin-like growth factor-I (IGF-I) receptor (Blakesley et al 1996). In addition, Yu and Roy (1999) reported that only a narrow range of low doses of insulin was maximally effective at promoting follicular development. Therefore, we treated bovine cortical pieces with graded doses of insulin or IGF-I. Surprisingly, IGF-I was deleterious to follicular survival, and the high dose of insulin present in ITS+ was the most effective in maintaining follicular health and growth. The deleterious effects of IGF were observed even in the presence of ITS+, and they could be ameliorated by addition of an antibody to IGF-I (Yang and Fortune 2002).

2.6 Summary and Conclusions

The activation of primordial follicles appears to be regulated by a myriad of factors, and the current evidence suggests that whether an individual follicle stays in the resting pool or initiates growth may depend on the balance of stimulatory and inhibitory factors impinging on the follicle at a particular point in time. Although it is particularly difficult to study the factors involved in the initiation of follicle growth in large mammals, my laboratory has developed two experimental models for studying the regulation of follicular activation and growth. In one model, using organ cultures of small pieces of ovarian cortex, almost all primordial follicles activate. This model may thus be useful for testing putative inhibitors of activation. In contrast, the second model, using grafts of ovarian cortical pieces beneath the CAM of chick embryos, provides an environment in which no or little activation occurs, and this situation may be used in the future to test potential stimulators of follicular activation. Our results thus far indicate that there may be significant species differences in the regulation of follicle activation and the initial growth of activated follicles. Although encouraging progress has been made in identifying potential regulators of follicular activation in rodents, there is much to be learned and this first critical transition of follicular development is still very poorly understood in larger mammals.

Acknowledgments. Drs. S.-A. Wandji, R.A. Cushman, S. Kito, A.K. Voss, V. Srsen, Mr. D.D. Byrd, and Mr. C. Murphy performed the studies reviewed in this manuscript. Their contributions and those of our collaborators, Drs. C.M. Wahl, J.J. Eppig, and P.W. Nathanielsz, are gratefully acknowledged. Financial support was provided by the NIH (R01HD35168 and F32HD08624) and the USDA (00–35203–9151).

References

Blakesley VA, Scimgeour A, Esposito D, Le Roith D (1996) Signaling via the insulin-like growth factor-I receptor: does it differ from insulin receptor signaling? Cytokine Growth Factor Rev 7:153–159

Braw-Tal R, Yossefi S (1997) Studies in vivo and in vitro on the initiation of follicle growth in the bovine ovary. J Reprod Fertil 109:165–171

Cushman RA, Gigli I, Wahl CM, Fortune JE (2001) Activation of mouse primordial follicles is inhibited in chorioallantoic membrane grafts. Biol Reprod 64[Suppl 1]:110

Cushman RA, Wahl CM, Fortune JE (2002) Bovine ovarian cortical pieces grafted to chick embryonic membranes: a model for studies on the activation of primordial follicles. Hum Reprod 17:48–52

Derrar N, Price CA, Sirard M-A (2000) Effect of growth factors and co-culture with ovarian medulla on the activation of primordial follicles in explants of bovine ovarian cortex. Theriogenology 54:587–598

DiClemente N, Ghaffari S, Pepinsky RB, Pieau C, Josso N, Cate RL, Vigier B (1992) A quantitative and interspecific test for biological activity of anti–Müllerian hormone: the fetal ovary aromatase assay. Development 114:721–727

Dissen GA, Romero C, Hirshfield AN, Ojeda SR (2001) Nerve growth factor is required for early follicular development in the mammalian ovary. Endocrinology 142:2078–2086

Durlinger ALL, Kramer P, Karels B, de Jong FH, Uilenbroek JTJ, Grootegoed JA, Themmen APN (1999) Control of primordial follicle recruitment by anti-Müllerian hormone in the mouse ovary. Endocrinology 140:5789–5796

Durlinger ALL, Gruijters MJG, Kramer P, Karels B, Ingraham HA, Nachtigal MW, Uilenbroek JTJ, Grootegoed JA, Themmen APN (2002) Anti-Müllerian hormone inhibits initiation of primordial follicle growth in the mouse ovary. Endocrinology 143:1076–1084

Eppig JJ, O'Brien MJ (1996) Development in vitro of mouse oocytes from primordial follicles. Biol Reprod 54:197–207

Fortune J, Kito S, Wandji S–A, Srsen V (1998) Activation of bovine and baboon primordial follicles in vitro. Theriogenology 49:441–449

Fortune JE, Kito S, Byrd DD (1999) Activation of primordial follicles in vitro. J Reprod Fertil Suppl 54:439–448

Fortune JE, Cushman RA, Wahl CM, Kito S (2000) The primordial to primary follicle transition. Mol Cell Endocrinol 163:53–60

Gougeon A (1996) Regulation of ovarian follicular development n primates: Facts and hypotheses. Endocrine Rev 17:121–155

Henricson B, Rajakoski E (1959) Studies of oocytogenesis in cattle. Cornell Vet 49:494–503

Herrmann G, Spanel-Borowski K (1998) A sparsely vascularized zone in the cortex of the bovine ovary. Anat Histol Embryol 27:143–146

Hirshfield AN (1991) Development of follicles in the mammalian ovary. Int Rev Cytol 124:43–101

Mayerhofer A, Dissen GA, Costa ME, Ojeda SR (1997) A role for neurotransmitters in early follicular development: induction of functional follicle-stimulating hormone receptors in newly formed follicles of the rat ovary. Endocrinology 138:3320–3329

McNatty KP, Fidler AE, Juengel JL, Quirke LD, Smith PR, Heath DA, Lundy T, O'Connell AO, Tisdall DJ (2000) Growth and paracrine factors regulating follicular formation and cellular function. Mol Cell Endocrinol 163:11–20

Nilsson E, Skinner MK (2001) Cellular interactions that control primordial follicle development and folliculogenesis. J Soc Gynecol Invest 8:S17–-S20

Picton HM (2001) Activation of follicle development: the primordial follicle. Theriogenology 55:1193–1210

Rawles M (1952) Transplantation of normal embryonic tissues in the chick embryo in biological research. Annals NY Acad Sci 55:302

Rudnick D (1944) Early history and mechanics of the chick blastoderm. Quart Rev Biol 197:187

Russe I (1983) Oogenesis in cattle and sheep. Bibl Anat 24:77–92

van Wagenen G, Simpson ME (1965) Embryology of the ovary and testis. *Homo sapiens* and *Macaca mulatta*. Yale University Press, New Haven

van Wezel IL, Rodgers RJ (1996) Morphological characterization of bovine primordial follicles and their environment in vivo. Biol Reprod 55:1003–1011

Wandji S-A, Srsen V, Voss AK, Eppig JJ, Fortune JE (1996) Initiation in vitro of growth of bovine primordial follicles. Biol Reprod 55:942–948

Wandji S-A, Srsen V, Nathanielsz PW, Eppig JJ, Fortune JE (1997) Initiation of growth of baboon primordial follicles in vitro. Hum Reprod 12:1993–2001

Yang MY, Fortune JE (2002) Insulin and IGF-I exert opposite effects on the activation of bovine primordial follicles in vitro. Biol Reprod 66[Suppl 1]:111

Yu N, Roy SK (1999) Development of primordial and prenatal follicles from undifferentiated somatic cells and oocytes in the hamster prenatal ovary in vitro: effect of insulin. Biol Reprod 61:1558–1567

3 Follicular Development and Apoptosis

H. Billig, E. Markström, E.C. Svensson, R. Shao, A. Friberg

3.1 Follicular Apoptosis ... 23
3.2 Mechanisms of Apoptosis ... 24
3.3 Models for Ovarian Apoptosis ... 28
3.4 Dependence on the Stage of Differentiation of the Follicle ... 28
3.5 Conclusions ... 37
References ... 37

3.1 Follicular Apoptosis

More than 99.9% of the ovarian follicles present at birth never reach ovulation. The most common fate of follicles is instead to undergo atresia, which has been shown to be mediated by a highly organised type of cell death called apoptosis or programmed cell death (Hsueh et al. 1994; Billig et al. 1996; Kaipia and Hsueh 1997). The final tuning of the large number of growing follicles to a single ovulatory follicle is primarily achieved by cell death of granulosa cells (Hsueh et al. 1994; Reynaud and Driancourt 2000).

The foetal human ovaries contain millions of germ cells, with a peak number observed at the fifth month of pregnancy (6.8×10^6 germ cells). Degeneration of germ cells occurs before formation of the ovarian follicles and thus regulates the number of primordial follicles endowed in the ovaries. Up until birth, the number of germ cells decreases dramatically, the number of germ cells enclosed in primordial follicles at birth being less than 20% of its peak number (Baker 1963).

The individual mammalian follicle consists of a central oocyte surrounded by somatic granulosa cell layers and outer layers of somatic theca cells. The maturation of ovarian follicles involves several sequential stages; initiation of growth of primordial follicles in the resting pool, growth of the follicles, selection of a dominant follicle, ovulation and finally luteinisation. The initiation of growth of resting primordial follicles, designated as initial recruitment (McGee and Hsueh 2000), is followed by growth, differentiation and atresia. When the follicle acquires an antral cavity, it becomes dependent on hormonal support from follicle stimulating hormone (FSH). During each reproductive cycle, increasing FSH concentrations recruit growing antral follicles. This rescue from degeneration has been suggested to be termed cyclic recruitment (McGee and Hsueh 2000). At the last stage in follicular development, the endogenous luteinizing hormone (LH) surge induces ovulation and corpus luteum formation. During the growth and development of follicles, atresia occurs at every stage of follicular development (Gougeon 1986), with one exception. The number of corpora lutea equals the number of follicles that respond to the LH surge, implying decreased apoptosis sensitivity at this final stage.

Follicular atresia is regulated by endocrine factors, such as FSH and LH, and by paracrine factors, including insulin-like growth factor (IGF)-I, epidermal growth factor (EGF), basic fibroblast growth factor (bFGF), activin and interleukin (IL)-1β. Atretogenic factors include tumour necrosis factor (TNF)-α, gonadotropin releasing hormone (GnRH), androgens, IL-6 and free radicals (Kaipia and Hsueh 1997). Granulosa cell apoptosis is an active cellular event, dependent on transcription as well as protein synthesis, since incubation in the presence of the transcription inhibitor actinomycin-D or the translation inhibitor cyclohexamide dose-dependently decreases the spontaneous apoptosis (Svanberg and Billig 1999).

3.2 Mechanisms of Apoptosis

Once the decision to die has been made, the execution of the apoptotic death requires co-ordinated activation and propagation of several subprogrammes (Hengartner 2000). Two families of important regulators of the apoptotic process are the caspase family and the Bcl-2 family

(Fig. 1). Caspases are thought of as the executioners of the apoptotic pathway (Hengartner 2000) and function as proteases cleaving after an aspartic acid residue. There are at least three mechanisms for caspase activation, including (1) processing by an upstream caspase, (2) association with cofactors and (3) cleavage induced by a high local concentration of caspases, associated to activated death receptors. Today, more than 100 substrates are known to be cleaved by caspases, including lamins, required for nuclear shrinking and budding, and cytoskeletal proteins such as fodrin and gelsolin, causing loss of overall cell shape (Hengartner 2000). Caspases are essential for shutting down the cellular machinery during apoptosis. For instance, granulosa cells from caspase-3 gene knockout mice demonstrate atretic follicles with lack of DNA degradation and aberrant morphology (Matikainen et al. 2001).

An important function of the caspases is to activate the endonuclease responsible for internucleosomal DNA fragmentation, one of the most frequently used hallmarks of apoptosis. the responsible endonuclease (caspase-activated DNase, CAD) and its inhibitory subunit (inhibitor of caspase-activated DNase, ICAD) are constantly expressed in the cells. Caspase-mediated cleavage of the inhibitory subunit results in release and activation of the endonuclease.

The Bcl-2 family of apoptotic regulators comprises both anti-apoptotic members, such as Bcl-2 and Bcl-X_L, and pro-apoptotic members, including Bax, Bid, Bik, BOD and Bcl-X_S. Members of the Bcl-2 family can both homodimerise and heterodimerise with several other family members, thereby regulating each other's activity. The essential function of the Bcl-2 family seems to be to regulate release of pro-apoptotic factors, in particular cytochrome *c*, from the mitochondrion into the cytosol (Antonsson and Martinou 2000). Many members of the Bcl-2 family have been isolated in the ovary, including BAD, Mcl-1 and Bok (Hsu and Hsueh 2000).

The mitochondrion is a crucial structure in the apoptotic machinery, harbouring several pro-apoptotic factors that are released to the cytoplasm upon a certain signal (Fig. 1). One of these factors is cytochrome *c*, forming a complex with an adapter protein termed Apaf-1 and a proform of caspase-9, which is required for caspase-9 activation in the cytosol. All these components are present in the follicular cells and Apaf-1 expression is suppressed by anti-apoptotic regulators like gonadotropins (Robles et al. 1999).

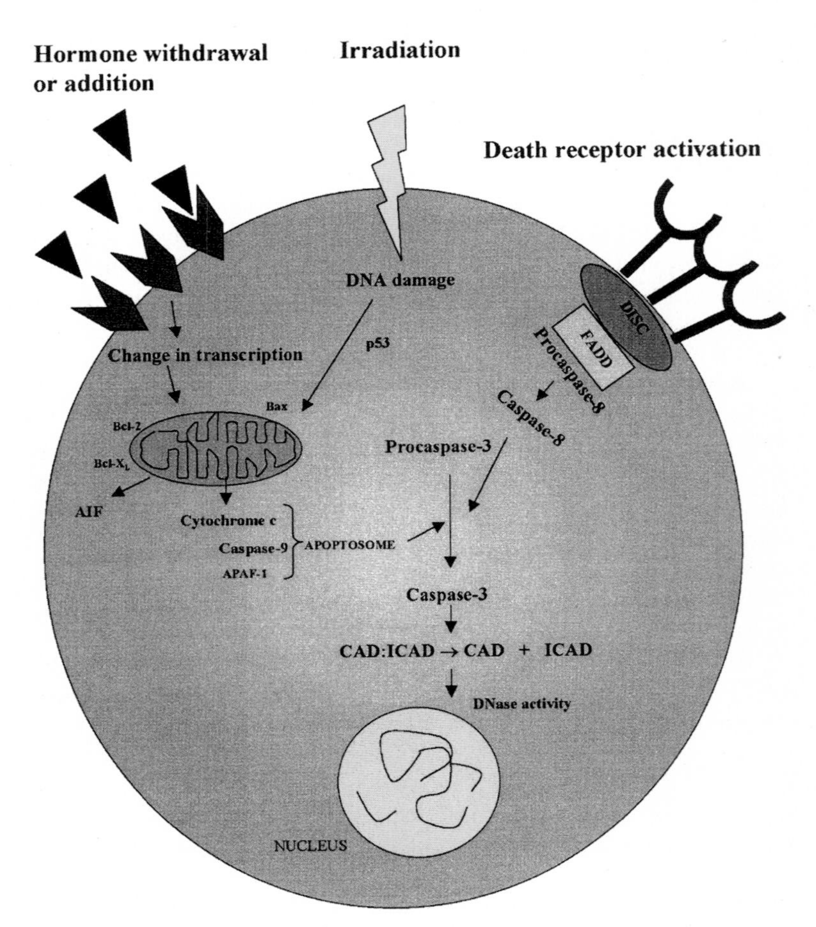

Fig. 1. Legend see p. 27

The question of how cytochrome *c* manages to cross the mitochondrial outer membrane is not yet solved, but the members of the Bcl-2 family are closely involved in the regulation of this process. Cytochrome *c* release is an almost universal event during apoptotic cell death. However, in some cases it is a very late event, like in apoptosis induced by death receptors, where the mitochondrial pathway is often bypassed and cytochrome *c* is released as a result of caspase activation (Scaffidi et al. 1998). In addition to cytochrome *c*, other pro-apoptotic factors are stored in the mitochondria and will be released upon induction of apoptosis. Examples include AIF (apoptosis inducing factor) and several pro-caspases.

After the apoptotic death, the remains of the cell are removed. On a molecular level, phosphatidylserine (PS) exposure on the outer side of the cell membrane is one signalling mechanism occurring in apoptotic cells (Fig. 1). In the ovary, SR-BI (scavenger receptor class B type I) on theca cells has been shown to mediate recognition and binding of apoptotic granulosa cells expressing PS on the cell surface (Svensson et al. 1999).

Fig. 1. Schematic overview of the apoptotic process in follicular granulosa cells, showing two major apoptotic pathways in mammalian cells. The *death receptor pathway* is triggered by members of the death receptor superfamily (e.g. CD95, tumour necrosis factor receptor I). Binding of ligand to these receptors causes receptor clustering and formation of a death inducing signalling complex (DISC). This complex recruits, via the adaptor molecule FADD (Fas-associated death domain protein), multiple procaspase-8 molecules, resulting in caspase-8 activation through induced proximity. The *mitochondrial pathway* is used extensively in response to extracellular apoptotic stimuli and internal insults such as DNA damage. These diverse response pathways converge on mitochondria, often through the activation of a pro-apoptotic member of the Bcl-2 family. Pro- and anti-apoptotic Bcl-2 family members meet at the surface of mitochondria, where they compete to regulate cytochrome c exit. If the pro-apoptotic side wins, an array of molecules is released from the mitochondrial compartment. Principal among these is cytochrome c, which associates with Apaf-1 and then procaspase-9 to form the apoptosome. The death receptor and mitochondrial pathways converge at the level of caspase-3 activation. Downstream of caspase-3, the apoptotic programme branches into a multitude of subprogrammes, among which internucleosomal DNA fragmentation is one. (Modified after Hengartner 2000)

3.3 Models for Ovarian Apoptosis

A range of stimuli can affect the decision of a cell to die. In the ovary, there are several specific regulators of apoptosis, including hormones, growth factors and cytokines (Fig. 1). Investigating ovarian apoptosis has the intrinsic problem of studying something that disappears. The apoptotic process ends with phagocytosis by surrounding cells, leaving no long-lasting traces for investigation. In addition, in the ovary the factors regulating apoptosis vary between follicle populations of different developmental stages, necessitating models where homogeneous cohorts of follicles can be isolated at specific stages.

Many models for studying follicular atresia have taken advantage of the fact that isolated follicles or granulosa cells undergo spontaneous apoptosis when cultured in the absence of serum (Tilly et al. 1992). Addition of survival or pro-apoptotic factors to the incubation medium can then affect the rate of this spontaneous apoptosis. Several rodent models have also been developed in order to isolate follicles at specific stages of development. For instance, diethylstilboestrol implants to hypophysectomised rats renders opportunity to study preantral and early antral follicles (Billig et al. 1993). Further differentiation can be achieved by sequential stimulation of the FSH and LH receptors of immature rats. In humans, the source of material is most often periovulatory granulosa cells collected from women undergoing oocyte aspiration prior to in vitro fertilisation.

3.4 Dependence on the Stage of Differentiation of the Follicle

Follicular atresia is a hormonally regulated process and different factors are affecting the decision to die at different developmental stages of the ovarian follicles. Although a number of locally produced growth factors have been demonstrated to affect follicle cell survival, the main physiological regulators of ovarian follicle survival are the gonadotropins. Most, if not all, of the factors presented in the literature as inhibitors of follicle atresia are regulated by FSH and LH. When the growing follicles reach the antral stage, they express receptors for FSH and become dependent on the FSH stimulation. Sufficient FSH concentrations are critical for survival of the follicles that have differentiated to the antral stage or further. During each reproductive cycle, the rise in FSH concentrations rescues developing follicles, a cyclic recruitment. LH, on the other hand, is important for follicles approaching ovulation and expressing the LH receptor. Blockage of the LH surge has been shown to result in massive atresia in rats (Braw and Tsafriri 1980). In the adult human ovary, the degree of atresia has been estimated to be highest in antral follicles larger than 5 mm in diameter (Gougeon 1986).

To understand the well-tuned balance of follicle growth and atresia, the differentiation-dependent regulation through follicular development has to be acknowledged.

3.4.1 Early Follicular Development

In primordial follicles, oocyte apoptosis is probably responsible for subsequent follicular degeneration. The phenomenon of oocyte apoptosis has recently been reviewed by Morita and Tilly (1999), and Reynaud and Driancourt (2000), describing the importance of, for instance, Kit–Kit ligand interaction and the growth factors EGF and bFGF in rodents. It has been reported that Kit–Kit ligand interaction is important for survival of primordial follicles in foetal as well as postnatal ovaries. Interaction probably prevents follicles from degeneration by rescuing the oocyte (Driancourt et al. 2000). Another oocyte-derived factor important for survival of small follicles is GDF-9 (growth and differentiation factor 9). Mice lacking GDF-9 have no follicle development beyond primary/early secondary stage (Dong et al. 1996).

The aryl hydrocarbon receptor (AhR) may be of importance for regulating the size of the pool of primordial germ cells. Ovaries collected from foetal mice and cultured in vitro showed a high degree of oocyte apoptosis. The number of non-apoptotic oocytes after culture of foetal ovaries from AhR-deficient mice was almost three times higher compared to wild-type (Robles et al. 2000). However, the endogenous ligand for AhR is presently unknown.

Preantral follicles are characterised by slow growth and there are distinct differences between human and rat follicles at this stage. Human follicles reach the preantral stage several months prior to ovulation, whereas rat follicles become preantral only a few days before ovulation.

Thus, although they are at the same morphological stage, there may be developmental differences between the preantral rat and human follicles (McGee 2000). Relatively little is known about regulation of survival of preantral follicles in rodents and humans compared to what is known about survival at later stages of development.

When isolated preantral follicles from 12- to 14-day-old rats are cultured in serum-free medium, there is a spontaneous onset of apoptosis in the granulosa cells, similar to what is seen in preovulatory follicles. At this early differentiation stage, FSH and its downstream mediator cAMP have no effect on apoptosis in cultured rat follicles (McGee et al. 1997a). However, this is not due to lack of FSH receptors, since FSH has the ability to enhance steroidogenic enzyme expression in preantral follicles (Dunkel et al. 1994; Rannikki et al. 1995). In contrast, both FSH and LH receptor stimulation are important for preantral rat follicle development in vivo (McGee et al. 1997b). This suggests that the gonadotropin effect is not direct on preantral follicles, but it is rather mediated via other gonadotropin-sensitive cells, such as cells in further differentiated follicles.

Locally produced survival factors for preantral follicles include keratinocyte growth factor (KGF). KGF is produced by theca cells in the ovary and receptors are found in granulosa cells. In cultured preantral rat follicles, KGF suppresses apoptosis and also promotes growth and differentiation (McGee et al. 1999). Likewise, FGF suppress apoptosis in cultured preantral rat follicles to the same extent (McGee et al. 1999). Other locally produced survival factors are oestrogens, which have been reported to decrease the degree of granulosa cell apoptosis in preantral follicles in vivo in hypophysectomised rats. Furthermore, this effect was abolished by treatment with testosterone (Billig et al. 1993).

Intracellular mediators for survival of preantral follicles include cGMP, but not cAMP. It has been reported that treatment of isolated rat preantral follicles with a cGMP analogue reduces the degree of apoptosis by as much as 75% (McGee et al. 1997a).

Dietary ascorbic acid (vitamin C) is known to affect fertility in humans. It was recently reported that addition of ascorbic acid to in vitro cultured mouse preantral follicles decrease the degree of apoptosis and increase the percentage of follicles that maintain basement membrane integrity (Murray et al. 2001).

Factors promoting growth of ovarian follicles, e.g. FSH and bFGF, also inhibit apoptosis, with some exceptions. For instance, MIS (Müllerian inhibitory substance) has recently been shown to promote growth of preantral rat follicles without affecting granulosa cell apoptosis or differentiation (McGee et al. 2001).

3.4.2 Late Follicular Development

During the normal reproductive cycle in humans and in rodents, the early antral follicular stage is probably the most critical stage of follicle development. Early antral follicles express receptors for FSH and become dependent on FSH stimulation for survival. Due to lack of FSH support, many follicles never pass this point in their development (see Hirshfield 1991).

Indeed, in isolated early antral rat follicles the gonadotropin FSH has been reported to be the most important survival factor. FSH was able to suppress apoptosis by up to 60%. This effect was partially reversed by addition of the IGF-binding protein IGFBP-3, indicating a mediatory role of IGF-I. On the other hand, LH receptor stimulation seems to have rather limited effect on survival of rat follicles at this stage (Chun et al. 1996).

Locally produced factors of importance for survival of isolated early antral rat follicles include IGF-I, EGF, bFGF, activin, and the cytokine IL-1β. GH (growth hormone) is unable to suppress apoptosis in cultured early antral follicles, despite inducing increased expression of IGF-I mRNA (Chun et al. 1996). Several of these locally produced factors are, however, more potent as survival factors in later stages of follicle development. For instance, IL-1β is threefold more effective in preventing apoptosis in preovulatory than in early antral follicles. Since IL-1β probably mediates its effects via receptors on theca cells, the higher degree of suppression in preovulatory follicles might be due to presence of more differentiated theca cells at that developmental stage (Chun et al. 1996). At the early antral stage, there is a differential effectiveness of the hormones/growth factors regulating survival of cultured rat follicles with FSHIGF-I, IL-1βLH, EGF, bFGF, activin>GH (Chun et al. 1996). As in preantral follicles, oestrogens have been shown to be of importance for survival of early antral follicles in vivo in rats (Billig et al.

1993). However, there is no report of oestrogens affecting survival of cultured follicles or granulosa cells.

3.4.3 Preovulatory Follicles

At the preovulatory stage of development the ovarian follicles express LH receptors and are able to respond to the soon-due LH surge. Both of the gonadotropins, FSH and LH, suppress the degree of apoptosis in isolated preovulatory rat follicles (Chun et al. 1994). Studies of cultured preovulatory rat follicles have shown that the suppression of apoptosis seen after treatment with gonadotropins may be partially mediated by endogenously produced IGF-I (Chun et al. 1994). At least three lines of evidence support this hypothesis (see Chun et al. 1994): (1) Addition of IGFBP-3 dose-dependently decreases the apoptosis suppressive effect of LH receptor stimulation, (2) higher levels of IGFBP-4 and -5 have been found in atretic human follicles than in healthy ones and (3) LH receptor stimulation results in increased IGF-I mRNA content in cultured preovulatory rat follicles. However, IGF-I has no effect in isolated granulosa cells from preovulatory follicles (Tilly et al. 1992), suggesting interaction with other follicular cells. Interestingly, the cytokine IL-1β has also been shown to mediate part of the apoptosis suppressive effects of gonadotropins in rats. Addition of an IL-1β receptor antagonist partially decreases the effect of gonadotropins (Chun et al. 1995). By itself, IL-1β suppresses apoptosis in cultured preovulatory follicles and simultaneous addition of an IL-1β antagonist reverses the effect. The effect of IL-1β is probably brought about by way of NO and cGMP generation (Chun et al. 1995).

The locally produced survival factors EGF and bFGF suppress apoptosis as effectively as gonadotropins in rat preovulatory follicles and isolated granulosa cells (Tilly et al. 1992). This effect is mediated through the tyrosine kinase pathway, since addition of the tyrosine kinase inhibitor genistein abolished the effect of EGF/bFGF. The EGF receptor has been shown to be upregulated by gonadotropins (Fujinaga et al. 1994), which probably explains the fact that there is no or minimal effect on apoptosis in preantral and early antral rat follicles (Tilly et al. 1992; McGee et al. 1997a). Transforming growth factor-α (TGF-α) is a structural and functional homologue of EGF that shares the same cell membrane receptor. Indeed, TGF-α mimics the effects of EGF in isolated preovulatory rat follicles (Tilly et al. 1992). KGF, a member of the FGF family, is also anti-apoptotic when added to cultured preovulatory rat follicles (McGee et al. 1999).

Another survival factor for cultured preovulatory rat follicles is insulin, since it has been reported that insulin decreases the apoptosis sensitivity in vitro (Chun et al. 1994). This effect is probably mediated by way of the IGF-I receptor and IGF-I has a stronger anti-apoptotic effect than insulin. Insulin has no effect on isolated preovulatory rat granulosa cells (Tilly et al. 1992), suggesting involvement of other ovarian cells. GH is also able to suppress apoptosis in cultured preovulatory rat follicles. Since the effect is inhibited by addition of IGFBP-3, it is probably mediated by IGF-I (Eisenhauer et al. 1995). In addition, it has been reported that mice overexpressing bovine GH have an increased number of healthy preovulatory follicles as well as a lower percentage of preovulatory follicles undergoing heavy apoptosis, compared to non-transgenic littermates (Danilovich et al. 2000). This is in contrast to earlier developmental stages, where GH does not affect apoptosis (Chun et al. 1996).

Intracellular mediators of preovulatory follicle survival include cAMP and cGMP. However, stimulation of protein kinase A or C signalling pathways in isolated rat granulosa cells has no effect on apoptosis (Tilly et al. 1992).

3.4.4 Periovulatory Follicles

Follicles that have survived up to the periovulatory stage are dependent on the endogenous LH surge. Blockage of the LH surge by hypophysectomy or pentobarbital treatment will cause the follicles to degenerate (Talbert et al. 1951; Braw and Tsafriri 1980). The decreased spontaneous apoptosis observed in isolated preovulatory rat follicles treated with human chorionic gonadotropin (hCG), in order to stimulate the LH receptor, has been suggested to be partially mediated by endogenous production of PACAP (pituitary adenylate cyclase-activating polypeptide). LH-induced suppression of follicular apoptosis is partly inhibited by co-treatment with a PACAP antagonist (Lee et al. 1999).

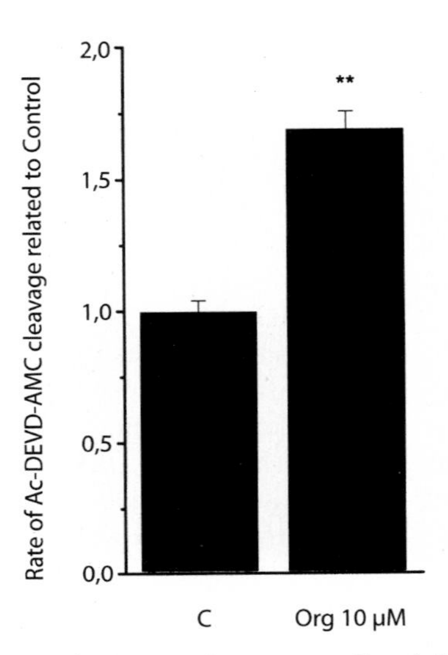

Fig. 2. Degree of apoptosis measured as caspase-3 activity in granulosa cells isolated from periovulatory follicles in hCG-treated rats after incubation in serum-free medium with or without addition of the progesterone receptor antagonist Org 31710 (10 μM). The fluorogenic substrate used was Ac-DEVD-AMC (**$p<0.01$; $n=3$). (Svensson et al. 2000)

After the LH surge the follicles are less susceptible to atresia than follicles at earlier stages, shown by a decreased apoptosis sensitivity in vitro (Svensson et al. 2000). The mechanism for this reduced sensitivity has been poorly studied, but recently progesterone has been shown to function as a regulator of apoptosis by way of its nuclear receptor (Fig. 2) in granulosa cells isolated from periovulatory follicles in rats (Svensson et al. 2000). Also, human periovulatory granulosa cells express the progesterone receptor (PR), and treatment in vitro with PR antagonists (Fig. 3) increases apoptosis (Makrigiannakis et al. 2000; Svensson et al. 2001). Non-nuclear receptor-mediated effects of progesterone have also been suggested. Progesterone has been attributed an apoptosis-inhibiting effect in immature and preovulatory (but not LH receptor-stimulated) rat granulosa cells via a g-aminobutyric acid (GABA) receptor-like receptor (Peluso and Pappalardo 1998). However, addition of GABA receptor antagonists (picrotoxin and bicuculline) as

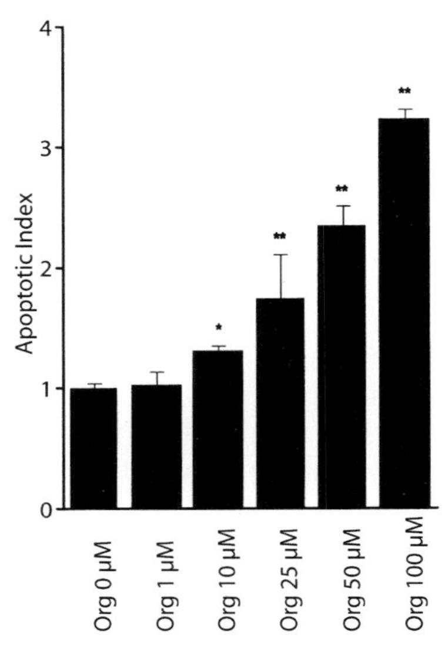

Fig. 3. Induction of apoptosis in human luteinizing granulosa cells in vitro by addition of the progesterone receptor antagonist Org 31710 to the culture medium. Addition of Org 31710 (1–100 μM) to the culture medium during 24-h incubation caused a dose-dependent increase in internucleosomal DNA fragmentation, quantified fluorospectrophotometrically (**$p<0.01$, *$p<0.05$ compared to Org 0 μM; $n=3$–9). (Svensson et al. 2001)

well as the GABA agonist muscimol to isolated granulosa cells from rat periovulatory follicles, did not influence the degree of apoptosis (Svensson et al. 2000).

Interestingly, expression of the nuclear PR is induced shortly after the LH surge in both rat and human granulosa cells, coinciding with the apoptosis-suppressive effects of progesterone. In rat granulosa cells, PR expression is transient (Park and Mayo 1991; Natraj and Richards 1993). Unlike in rat, where PR is not expressed in the corpus luteum, the PR in humans persists in luteinizing granulosa cells in the corpus luteum during early pregnancy (Press and Greene 1988; Iwai et al. 1990). Granulosa cells in non-dominant human ovarian follicles do not express PR (Iwai et al. 1990).

Mice lacking both isoforms of the PR (A and B) are anovulatory, strengthening the probability for direct effects of progesterone in the ovary (Lydon et al. 1995, 1996). Lately, mice lacking only the A isoform of the receptor have been reported to have decreased ovulation after stimulation (Mulac-Jericevic et al. 2000), whereas mice lacking only the B isoform are fertile with normal litter sizes (Mulac-Jericevic et al. 2001). It has also been reported that addition of progestins augment gonadotropin-stimulated progesterone production by cultured rat granulosa cells (Fanjul et al. 1983).

The progesterone–PR complex functions as a transcription factor, making it possible to study gene expression to learn more about PR-mediated effects in the periovulatory follicles. Since granulosa cell apoptosis is dependent on transcription (Svanberg and Billig 1999), this may include, in addition to other effects, transcriptional changes that regulate apoptosis. In recent years, several genes have been identified as PR-regulated in granulosa cells during the periovulatory interval, including PACAP and its receptor PAC_1 (Ko et al. 1999; Ko and Park-Sarge 2000), and the proteases ADAMTS-1 and cathepsin L (Robker et al. 2000). In an attempt to demonstrate PR-regulated genes, we have treated periovulatory rat granulosa cells with PR blockers in vitro and studied the global mRNA expression with DNA microarray techniques. Preliminary data suggest that more than 3,000 genes could be detected and the expression of almost 100 genes were changed after treatment with PR-blocker.

Groups of regulated genes were identified as belonging to metabolic or functional pathways, including steroid metabolism and transport, angiogenesis, follicular rupture and stress responses. These preliminary data open the possibility that not only the progesterone receptor is of importance for regulation of apoptosis in periovulatory follicles, but also the metabolic regulation progesterone metabolism seems to harbour several regulatory checkpoints with implications on follicular development and demise.

3.5 Conclusions

Follicular development, characterised by a high rate of proliferation and apoptosis, is a tightly regulated process that is dependent on a balance between local ovarian growth factors and circulating hormones. However, the diminishing number of follicles in each developmental stage suggests that the control of follicular survival or atresia cannot be the same at each stage. Indeed, as discussed above, all follicles are not alike. Susceptibility to undergo apoptosis, as well as the regulators of follicle survival, changes during development.

References

Antonsson B, Martinou JC (2000) The Bcl-2 protein family Experimental Cell Res 256 50–57

Baker TG (1963) A quantitative and cytological study of germ cells in human ovaries. Proceedings of the Royal Society of London. Biol Sci 158 417–433

Billig H, Furuta I, Hsueh AJ (1993) Estrogens inhibit and androgens enhance ovarian granulosa cell apoptosis. Endocrinology 133:2204–2212

Billig H, Chun SY, Eisenhauer K, Hsueh AJ (1996) Gonadal cell apoptosis: hormone-regulated cell demise. Hum Reprod Update 2:103–117

Braw RH, Tsafriri A (1980) Follicles explanted from pentobarbitone-treated rats provide a model for atresia. J Reprod Fertil 59:259–265

Chun SY, Billig H, Tilly JL, Furuta I, Tsafriri A, Hsueh AJ (1994) Gonadotropin suppression of apoptosis in cultured preovulatory follicles: mediatory role of endogenous insulin-like growth factor I. Endocrinology 135:1845–1853

Chun SY, Eisenhauer KM, Kubo M, Hsueh AJ (1995) Interleukin-1 beta suppresses apoptosis in rat ovarian follicles by increasing nitric oxide production. Endocrinology 136:3120–3127

Chun SY, Eisenhauer KM, Minami S, Billig H, Perlas E, Hsueh AJ (1996) Hormonal regulation of apoptosis in early antral follicles: follicle-stimulating hormone as a major survival factor. Endocrinology 137:1447–1456

Danilovich NA, Bartke A, Winters TA (2000) Ovarian follicle apoptosis in bovine growth hormone transgenic mice. Biol of Reprod 62:103–107

Dong J, Albertini DF, Nishimori K, Kumar TR, Lu N, Matzuk MM (1996) Growth differentiation factor-9 is required during early ovarian folliculogenesis. Nature 383:531–535

Driancourt MA, Reynaud K, Cortvrindt R, Smitz J (2000) Roles of KIT and KIT LIGAND in ovarian function. Rev Reprod 5:143–152

Dunkel L, Tilly JL, Shikone T, Nishimori K, Hsueh AJ (1994) Follicle-stimulating hormone receptor expression in the rat ovary: increases during prepubertal development and regulation by the opposing actions of transforming growth factors beta and alpha. Biol Reprod 50:940–948

Eisenhauer KM, Chun SY, Billig H, Hsueh AJ (1995) Growth hormone suppression of apoptosis in preovulatory rat follicles and partial neutralization by insulin-like growth factor binding protein. Biol Reprod 53:13–20

Fanjul LF, Ruiz de Galarreta CM, Hsueh AJ (1983) Progestin augmentation of gonadotropin-stimulated progesterone production by cultured rat granulosa cells. Endocrinol 112:405–407

Fujinaga H, Yamoto M, Shikone T, Nakano R (1994) FSH and LH up-regulate epidermal growth factor receptors in rat granulosa cells. J Endocrinol 140:171–177

Gougeon A (1986) Dynamics of follicular growth in the human: a model from preliminary results. Hum Reprod 1:81–87

Hengartner MO (2000) The biochemistry of apoptosis. Nature 407:770–776

Hirshfield AN (1991) Development of follicles in the mammalian ovary. Int Rev Cytol 124:43–101

Hsu SY, Hsueh AJ (2000) Tissue-specific Bcl-2 protein partners in apoptosis: An ovarian paradigm. Physiol Rev 80:593–614

Hsueh AJ, Billig H, Tsafriri A (1994) Ovarian follicle atresia: a hormonally controlled apoptotic process. Endocrine Rev 15:707–724

Iwai T, Nanbu Y, Iwai M, Taii S, Fujii S, Mori T (1990) Immunohistochemical localization of oestrogen receptors and progesterone receptors in the human ovary throughout the menstrual cycle. Virchows Arch A Pathol Anat Histopathol 417:369–375

Kaipia A, Hsueh AJ (1997) Regulation of ovarian follicle atresia. Ann Rev Physiol 59:349–363

Ko C, Park-Sarge OK (2000) Progesterone receptor activation Mediates LH-induced type-I pituitary adenylate cyclase activating polypeptide receptor (PAC(1)) gene expression in rat granulosa cells. Biochem Biophys Res Commun 277:270–279

Ko C, In YH, Park-Sarge OK (1999) Role of progesterone receptor activation in pituitary adenylate cyclase activating polypeptide gene expression in rat ovary. Endocrinology 140:5185–5194

Lee J, Park HJ, Choi HS, Kwon HB, Arimura A, Lee BJ, Choi WS, Chun SY (1999) Gonadotropin stimulation of pituitary adenylate cyclase-activating polypeptide (PACAP) messenger ribonucleic acid in the rat ovary and the role of PACAP as a follicle survival factor. Endocrinology 140:818–826

Lydon JP, DeMayo FJ, Funk CR, Mani SK, Hughes AR, Montgomery CA Jr, Shyamala G, Conneely OM, O'Malley BW (1995) Mice lacking progesterone receptor exhibit pleiotropic reproductive abnormalities. Genes Dev 9:2266–2278

Lydon JP, DeMayo FJ, Conneely OM, O'Malley BW (1996) Reproductive phenotypes of the progesterone receptor null mutant mouse. J Steroid Biochem Mol Biol 56:67–77

Makrigiannakis A, Coukos G, Christofidou-Solomidou M, Montas S, Coutifaris C (2000) Progesterone is an autocrine/paracrine regulator of human granulosa cell survival in vitro. Ann NY Acad Sci 900:16–25

Matikianen T, Perez GI, Zheng TS, Kluzak TS, Rueda BR, Flavell RA, Tilly JL (2001) Caspase-3 gene knockout defines cell lineage specificity for programmed cell death signaling in the ovary. Endocrinology 142:2468–2467

McGee EA (2000) The regulation of apoptosis in preantral ovarian follicles. Biol Signals Recept 9:81–86

McGee EA, Hsueh AJ (2000) Initial and cyclic recruitment of ovarian follicles. Endocrine Rev 21:200–214

McGee E, Spears N, Minami S, Hsu SY, Chun SY, Billig H, Hsueh AJ (1997a) Preantral ovarian follicles in serum-free culture: suppression of apoptosis after activation of the cyclic guanosine 3′,5′-monophosphate pathway and stimulation of growth and differentiation by follicle-stimulating hormone. Endocrinology 138:2417–2424

McGee EA, Perlas E, LaPolt PS, Tsafriri A, Hsueh AJ (1997b) Follicle-stimulating hormone enhances the development of preantral follicles in juvenile rats. Biol Reprod 57:990–998

McGee EA, Chun SY, Lai S, He Y, Hsueh AJ (1999) Keratinocyte growth factor promotes the survival, growth, and differentiation of preantral ovarian follicles. Fertil Steril 71:732–738

McGee EA, Smith R, Spears N, Nachtigal MW, Ingraham H, Hsueh AJ (2001) Mullerian inhibitory substance induces growth of rat preantral ovarian follicles. Biol Reprod 64:293–298

Morita Y, Tilly JL (1999) Oocyte apoptosis: like sand through an hourglass. Develop Biol 213 1–17

Mulac-Jericevic B, Mullinax RA, DeMayo FJ, Lydon JP, Conneely OM (2000) Subgroup of reproductive functions of progesterone mediated by progesterone receptor-B isoform. Science 289:1751–1754

Mulac-Jericevic B, Mullinax RA, Conneely OM (2001) Phenotypic analysis of mice lacking progesterone receptor B isoform. The Endocrine Society's 83rd Annual Meeting (Abstract P1–P67)

Murray AA, Molinek MD, Baker SJ, Kojima FN, Smith MF, Hillier SG, Spears N (2001) Role of ascorbic acid in promoting follicle integrity and survival in intact mouse ovarian follicles in vitro. Reproduction 121:89–96

Natraj U, Richards JS (1993) Hormonal regulation, localization, and functional activity of the progesterone receptor in granulosa cells of rat preovulatory follicles. Endocrinology 133:761–769

Park OK, Mayo KE (1991) Transient expression of progesterone receptor messenger RNA in ovarian granulosa cells after the preovulatory luteinizing hormone surge. Mol Endocrinol 5:967–978

Peluso JJ, Pappalardo A (1998) Progesterone mediates its anti-mitogenic and anti-apoptotic actions in rat granulosa cells through a progesterone-binding protein with gamma aminobutyric acidA receptor-like features. Biol Reprod 58:1131–1137

Press MF, Greene GL (1988) Localization of progesterone receptor with monoclonal antibodies to the human progestin receptor. Endocrinology 122:1165–1175

Rannikki AS, Zhang FP, Huhtaniemi IT (1995) Ontogeny of follicle-stimulating hormone receptor gene expression in the rat testis and ovary. Mol Cell Endocrinol 107:199–208

Reynaud K, Driancourt MA (2000) Oocyte attrition. Mol Cell Endocrinol 163:101–108

Robker RL, Russell DL, Espey LL, Lydon JP, O'Malley BW, Richards JS (2000) Progesterone-regulated genes in the ovulation process: ADAMTS-1 and cathepsin L proteases. Proc Natl Acad Sci USA 97:4689–4694

Robles R, Tao X-J, Trbovich AM, Maravei DV, Nahum R, Perez GI, Tilly KL, Tilly JL (1999) Localization, regulation and possible consequences of apoptotic protease-activating factor-1 (Apaf-1) expression in granulosa cells of the mouse ovary. Endocrinology 140:2641–2644

Robles R, Morita Y, Mann KK, Perez GI, Yang S, Matikainen T, Sherr DH, Tilly JL (2000) The aryl hydrocarbon receptor, a basic helix-loop-helix transcription factor of the PAS gene family, is required for normal ovarian germ cell dynamics in the mouse. Endocrinology 141:450–453

Scaffidi C, Fulda S, Srinivasan A, Friesen C, Li F, Tomaselli KJ, Debatin KM, Krammer PH, Peter ME (1998) Two CD95 (APO-1/Fas) signaling pathways. EMBO J 17:1675–1687

Svanberg B, Billig H (1999) Isolation of differentially expressed mRNA in ovaries after estrogen withdrawal in hypophysectomized diethylstilbestrol-treated rats: increased expression during apoptosis. J Endocrinol 163 309–316

Svensson PA, Johnson MS, Ling C, Carlsson LM, Billig H, Carlsson B (1999) Scavenger receptor class B type I in the rat ovary: possible role in high density lipoprotein cholesterol uptake and in the recognition of apoptotic granulosa cells. Endocrinology 140:2494–2500

Svensson EC, Markström E, Andersson M, Billig H (2000) Progesterone receptor-mediated inhibition of apoptosis in granulosa cells isolated from rats treated with human chorionic gonadotropin. Biol Reprod 63:1457–1464

Svensson EC, Markstrom E, Shao R, Andersson M, Billig H (2001) Progesterone receptor antagonists Org 31710 and RU 486 increase apoptosis in human periovulatory granulosa cells. Fertil Steril 76:1225–1231

Talbert GB, Meyer RK, McShan WH (1951) Effect of hypophysectomy at the beginning of proestrus on maturing follicles in the ovary of the rat. Endocrinology 49:687–694

Tilly JL, Billig H, Kowalski KI, Hsueh AJ (1992) Epidermal growth factor and basic fibroblast growth factor suppress the spontaneous onset of apoptosis in cultured rat ovarian granulosa cells and follicles by a tyrosine kinase-dependent mechanism. Mol Endocrinol 6:1942–1950

4 Delivery of the Oocyte from the Follicle to the Oviduct: A Time of Vulnerability

J.S. Richards

4.1 Overview: Ovulation a Time of Vulnerability 43
4.2 The Essential Role of the Cumulus Cells in Ovulation 45
4.3 How Do Theca Cells Control the Ovulation Process? 48
4.4 Granulosa Cells Control Specific Steps in the Ovulation Process .. 49
4.5 Regulated Expression of Wnts and Frizzleds in the Ovary 53
4.6 Summary 55
References 55

4.1 Overview: Ovulation a Time of Vulnerability

Ovulation is the complex process by which the follicle-enclosed oocyte is released from the ovary for transfer to the oviduct where it can be fertilized. To prepare for ovulation, the ovary undergoes a series of closely regulated events that are controlled by hormones, growth factors, and intrafollicular regulatory molecules. Small follicles must mature to the preovulatory stage during which time the oocyte, granulosa cells, and theca cells acquire specific functional characteristics. The oocyte becomes competent to undergo meiosis. Granulosa cells acquire the ability to produce estrogens and respond to luteinizing hormone (LH) via the LH receptor. Theca cells begin to synthesize increasing amounts of androgens that serve as substrates for the aromatase enzyme in the granulosa cells (for review, Eppig 1991; Richards 1994). Remarkably, many events are spatially restricted to specific microenvironments

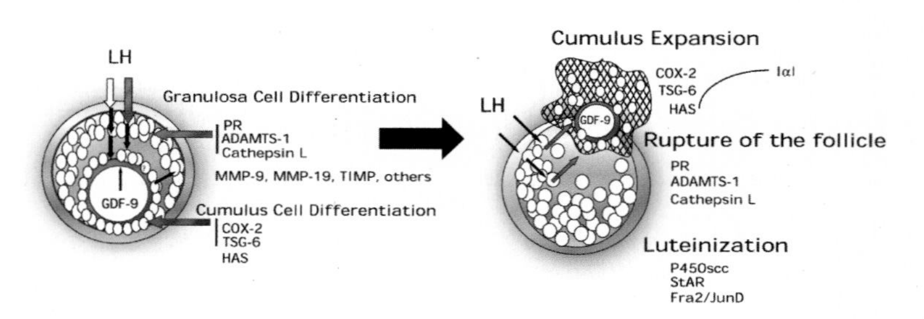

Fig. 1. LH-regulated genes that impact ovulation. The *LH* surge induces genes that control cumulus cell expansion [cyclooxygenase-2, *COX-2* and hyaluronic acid (HA) synthase, *HAS*] as well as those obligatory for follicle rupture (progesterone receptor, *PR*). LH induction of COX-2 in cumulus cells may be direct via LH receptors or indirect via impacting the GDF-9 signaling pathway. Expression of COX-2, production of prostaglandins (*PGE2*) and activation of EP2 receptors appear to be required for the expression of tumor necrosis stimulated genes-6, TSG-6, an HA-binding protein. Dissolution of the basement membrane allows entry of inter-α-inhibitor, IαI, another HA-binding protein that covalently couples to HA providing stability for the extracellular matrix. Expression of PR in granulosa cells is obligatory for the expression of two novel proteases, a disintegrin and metalloproteinase with thrombospondin-like repeats, ADAMTS-1 and cathepsin L in ovulating follicles. The exact roles of these two proteases in the ovulation process remain to be clearly defined. Substrates for ADAMTS-1 include versican and brevican as well as other proteins. Substrates for cathepsin L can be either lysosomal or extracellular matrix proteins such as laminin and fibronectin. Events of ovulation must occur before the granulosa cells and theca cells become fully differentiated, non-dividing luteal cells. (Adapted from Richards 2001; see also Richards et al. 2002a,b)

within the follicle or surrounding interstitial compartments to allow successful expulsion of the cumulus–oocyte complex (COC) from the ruptured follicle (Hess et al. 1999; Hizaki et al. 1999; Sato et al. 2001; Zhou et al. 2001) (Fig. 1). Failure of any one of these events prevents ovulation. Oocytes become entrapped in follicles or corpora lutea and eventually degenerate. In essence, ovulation is a unique biological event that is obligatory for reproductive success of all species. Our understanding of this process is critical for designing better ways to improve and regulate fertility. This text describes some recent results that document the specific roles of the granulosa cells in directing successful rupture of the follicle as well as the cumulus cells in synthesizing a matrix obligatory for the release of the oocyte from the follicle and its transport into the oviduct.

4.2 The Essential Role of the Cumulus Cells in Ovulation

The oocyte is surrounded by a specialized group of cells called the cumulus cells. These cells are directly in contact with the oocyte and comprise a specialized functional unit during follicular growth. In response to the ovulatory LH surge, the cumulus cells begin to synthesize special extracellular matrix proteins that are essential for the process known as cumulus expansion (Eppig 1979; Salustri et al. 1999). The pioneering studies of many investigators have shown that the matrix is formed by at least three major components: hyaluronic acid (HA; Eppig 1979; Hess et al. 1999; Salustri et al. 1999) and at least two HA-binding proteins. The HA-binding proteins are tumor-necrosis factor stimulated gene TSG-6 (Fulop et al. 1997; Yoshioka et al. 2000) and the serum-derived inter-α-inhibitor (IαI), also known as inter-α-trypsin inhibitor (ITI) or *s*erum-derived *h*yaluronic *a*cid binding *p*rotein (SHAP; Hess et al. 1999; Sato et al. 2001; Zhou et al. 2001). HA is a high-molecular-weight (several million daltons), linear, unbranched glycosaminoglycan. In the ovary, HA is produced by the cumulus cells and granulosa cells adjacent to the antrum (Eppig 1979, 1991; Salustri et al. 1999). Expansion occurs only when IαI enters the follicle or when serum is added to cumulus-oocyte complexes (COC) to stabilize the matrix by covalent coupling to the heavy chain (HC) of IαI (Hess et al. 1999; Salustri et al. 1999). The cumulus-derived matrix may also contain other factors such as the proteoglycans brevican and versican (MacArthur et al. 2000).

The LH surge initiates cumulus expansion by inducing the expression of specific genes. One of these is cyclooxygenase-2 (COX-2) the rate-limiting enzyme in the synthesis of prostaglandins such as prostaglandin E_2 (PGE2) (Joyce et al. 2001; Sirois et al. 1992). PGE2 binds to a specific G-protein coupled receptor, EP2 thereby regulating cAMP levels in cumulus cells. Ovulation is impaired in mice null for COX-2 (Dinchuk et al. 1995; Morham et al. 1995) and EP2 (Hizaki et al. 1999; Tilley et al. 1999). In each mutant mouse, the COCs within preovulatory follicles fail to undergo cumulus expansion in response to LH (Davis et al. 1999). Ovulation and cumulus expansion can be restored in the COX-2 mice by exogenous administration of PGE2 or interleukin (IL)-1β (Davis et al. 1999) indicating that prostaglandins and other signaling pathways are obligatory for both events. These observations provide clear evidence that one critical site for PGE2 action in the ovulating follicle is the COC.

The LH surge also leads to the induction of HA synthase-2 (HAS-2) which catalyzes the production of HA (Weigel et al. 1997) and TSG-6, which is a HA-binding protein (Lee et al. 1992; Fulop et al. 1997; Yoshioka et al. 2000). TSG-6 appears to be one target of PGE2 action in cumulus cells, since the expression of this gene is selectively reduced in the cumulus cells (but not granulosa cells) of COX-2- *and* EP2-null mice (S. Ochsner et al., manuscript submitted). Notably, TSG-6 message is induced within 4 h of LH/human chorionic gonadotropin (hCG) stimulation of preovulatory follicles. At that time it is present in both cumulus cells and granulosa cells adjacent to the antral cavity. By 12 h, TSG-6 remains expressed only in cumulus cells of ovulating follicles. TSG-6 is absent from cumulus cells at all time points in the COX-2- and EP2-null mice (S. Ochsner et al., manuscript submitted). These results indicate that PGE2 regulates expression of TSG-6 within the cumulus microenvironment and that TSG-6 may play some critical role in expansion of the matrix. Both TSG-6 and HA are expressed several hours prior to any visible physical expansion of the matrix (i.e., dispersion of the cumulus cells away from the oocyte). This suggests that the presence of these molecules is not sufficient for matrix formation or the movement of cumulus cells away from the oocyte.

One factor that has been shown to be essential for cumulus cell expansion is the serum-derived protein, IαI. Mice deficient for IαI (bikunin null mice) also fail to ovulate and exhibit impaired cumulus expansion (Sato et al. 2001; Zhou et al. 2001). Ovulation can be restored in the IαI-deficient mice by adding serum (Sato et al. 2001; Zhou et al. 2001). IαI is normally excluded from follicular fluid because of its size and the avascular nature of the granulosa cell layer. It enters upon dissolution of the basal lamina during LH-induced ovulation (Hess et al. 1999). IαI is composed of several subunits: the light chain (LC) known as bikunin, which is covalently associated with the heavy chains (HC) via a chondroitin-sulfate moiety. In the presence of HA, IαI undergoes a substitution reaction in which the HC (SHAP) is covalently bound to HA releasing the bikunin (Sato et al. 2001). The high degree of covalent linkage between the heavy chains and HA in the cumulus-oocyte matrix is unprecedented (Chen et al. 1996), and suggests that the enzyme activity controlling this process is elevated within the follicle. Indeed, studies by Larsen and colleagues have shown high activity of the HC–HA conversion process in mural granulosa cells (Chen et al. 1996). Although the enzymatic activity that catalyzes the covalent linkage to HA is essential, the biochemical identity of this converting enzyme is not yet known. Nor is it known if the enzyme is hormonally regulated in the mural granulosa cells. Such a condition would also be an important factor in controlling matrix formation. Recently, TSG-6 has also been reported to form a complex with the HC of IαI in the ovary (Mukhopadhyay et al. 2001). Collectively these observations indicate that HA and IαI, as well as COX-2-/PGE2-/EP2-induced gene products (TSG-6 and others?) are critical for cumulus–oocyte matrix formation or cumulus cell differentiation; lack of any one of these factors precludes expansion.

The molecular mechanisms by which LH induces expression of HAS-2, COX-2, and TSG-6 genes remains to be clearly defined. LH may act directly via LH receptors present on cumulus cells (although this possibility is controversial) or indirectly via the activation of other signaling events in the follicle. The latter has recently gained credence since the previously unknown soluble oocyte-derived factor that is essential for cumulus expansion (Eppig 1991; Salustri et al. 1999) has been provisionally identified as growth differentiation factor-9, GDF-9 (Elvin et al. 1999). In cultures of rodent granulosa cells, GDF-9-enriched medium can induce the expression of both HA and COX-2 (Elvin et al. 1999). In vivo, however, GDF-9 is expressed in oocytes beginning at the small primary follicle stage and continues in the oocyte after ovulation. If GDF-9 is the stimulatory factor, this raises the dilemma of why the expression of HA and COX-2 is restricted to ovulating follicles; i.e., those stimulated by the LH surge. One possible scenario that would link the obligatory requirement of LH action with that of the soluble oocyte-derived factor (i.e., GDF-9) is that this factor may need to be modified before it becomes activated. GDF-9, like other members of the TGF-β family, is synthesized as a pro-peptide and therefore it is likely present as a latent factor at the surface of the oocyte–cumulus cell junctions, possibly attached to proteoglycans (Park et al. 2000). Induction by LH of a specific protease may be necessary to activate and/or release GDF-9, thereby allowing it to interact with cellular receptors and induce HAS-2 and COX-2 in cumulus cells. Full resolution of the pathways by which LH induces COX-2 in granulosa cells versus cumulus cells will necessitate stage-specific knockouts of GDF-9. Knockouts of TSG-6 are also needed to convincingly show a role for this protein in cumulus expansion in vivo (Fig. 1).

4.3 How Do Theca Cells Control the Ovulation Process?

Theca cells are the critical source of androgens within the preovulatory follicles. However, the specific ovulatory role of the theca cells is not well defined. Although one might predict that theca cells would be the source of critical proteases necessary to disrupt the basal lamina or surrounding matrices in the interstitial layer, evidence for this has not yet emerged. Matrix metalloproteinase (MMP)2 is expressed exclusively in the theca cells of preantral, preovulatory, and ovulating follicles (Lui et al. 1998); however, mice null for MMP2 are fertile (Werb 1989). Other MMPs and their inhibitors (tissue inhibitors of metalloproteinase, TIMPs) exhibit more complex expression patterns, and mice null for many of these genes remain fertile (Curry and Osteen 2001). Based on the regulated expression of several aldo-keto reductase enzymes in the theca cells, it is possible that they act more as a protective shield to ensure that toxic levels (Richards et al. 2002b) of compounds do not reach the granulosa cells or the oocyte at an inopportune time.

These changes may serve also to protect the theca cells themselves and the ovary in general from exposure to toxic compounds.

4.4 Granulosa Cells Control Specific Steps in the Ovulation Process

First of all, granulosa cells of preovulatory follicles are the major producers of estradiol (derived from theca cell androgens via aromatase) that is the trigger for the LH surge. The LH surge rapidly turns off genes that control granulosa cells functions in growing follicles, such as the cell-cycle regulator cyclin D2 (Robker and Richards 1998a,b). At the same time, the LH surge induces genes in granulosa cells that are obligatory for ovulation as well as luteinization (Richards 1994; Richards et al. 2000, 2002b). The events associated with ovulation must occur before the events of luteinization are complete or oocytes become entrapped in a functional corpus luteum. Timing is of the essence and requires specific changes in granulosa cell function.

Many transcription factors are induced by the LH surge in granulosa cells of preovulatory follicles. These include early growth regulatory factor-1 (Egr-1; Espey et al. 2000a), CAAT enhancer binding protein beta [C/EBPβ; (Sirois and Richards 1993)] and progesterone receptor (PR; Natraj and Richards 1993; Park and Mayo 1991). Like COX-2, each of these components of the ovulatory process is induced rapidly, but is expressed only transiently, with peak levels of message and protein observed approximately 4–6 h after the LH surge. Each of these transcription factors appears to be involved in the functional activity of granulosa cells of ovulating follicles as revealed by knockout studies (for review see Richards et al. 1998, 2000; Richards et al. 2002b). Other transcription factors such as the activator protein-1 (AP-1) family members (e.g., Fra2 and JunD) are induced rapidly by the LH surge but then remain elevated in the non-dividing terminally differentiated granulosa cells during the postovulatory luteal phase (Sharma and Richards 2000).

PR is a member of the nuclear receptor superfamily and regulates the numerous functions in reproductive tissues, including the uterus, mammary gland, and ovary. In the ovary, LH rapidly and selectively induces PR in mural granulosa cells of preovulatory follicles (Park and Mayo 1991; Natraj and Richards 1993; Robker et al. 2000). The molecular mechanisms by which LH acts to induce PR are not yet entirely clear. In contrast to other tissues, strong evidence for a role of the estrogen receptor (ER) is lacking. Estradiol (E) alone does not induce PR in intact cells in vivo or in vitro (Natraj and Richards 1993). Nor does E induce activity of PR-promoter luciferase constructs transfected into granulosa cells (Clemens et al. 1998; Sharma and Richards 2002). Although ovulation is impaired in the ERαKO mouse, it can be restored fully by controlling pituitary secretion of LH (Couse et al. 1999; Couse and Korach 1999). Two regions of the PR promoter previously thought to be involved in mediating LH induction of this gene, namely the GC-rich region of the distal promoter and the ERE3 site of the proximal promoter (Clemens et al. 1998) also do not seem to be required in the context of the intact promoter (Sharma and Richards 2002). Deletion or mutation of these regions in the context of the intact murine promoter does not alter functional activity of a luciferase reporter construct when transfected into primary cultures of granulosa cells. Transactivation of the PR promoter in these cells appears to utilize a specific region that is currently being analyzed (Sharma and Richards 2002).

What is unequivocal is that mice null for PR fail to ovulate even when stimulated by exogenous hormones (Lydon et al. 1995; Robker et al. 2000). These findings support other studies that implicated progesterone as a key player in the ovulatory process (Lydon et al. 1995; Rose et al. 1999; Pall et al. 2000). More specifically, mice null for PRA but not PRB exhibit impaired ovulation, indicating a sub-type specificity of PR action in the ovulation process (Mulac-Jericevic et al. 2000; Conneely et al. 2001). Despite the failure of ovulation to occur in PRKO/PRAKO mice, the expression of COX-2, cumulus expansion, and luteinization proceed normally (Robker et al. 2000). Thus, the cumulus microenvironment is functional and signaling events that mediate granulosa cell differentiation in response to LH are intact. Recently, two targets of PR action that belong to two distinct classes of proteases have been identified. These are ADAMTS-1, a disintegrin and metalloproteinase with thrombospondin-like repeats, that is known as METH-1 in human (Vazquez et al. 1999; Espey et al. 2000b) and cathepsin L (Robker et al. 2000). Expression of ADAMTS-1 and cathepsin L mRNA is markedly reduced in granulosa cells of PR-null mice.

LH induces ADAMTS-1 selectively in granulosa cells and cumulus cells with peak levels of mRNA and protein being expressed 8–12 h after exposure of ovaries to an ovulatory dose of gonadotropin (Espey et al. 2000b; Robker et al. 2000). Therefore, the highest levels of ADAMTS-1 transcription occur after the peak of PR expression but before ovulation, which is usually observed at 14–16 h after exposure to ovulatory hormones in mice and rats. Quite significantly, there are clear data to show that the induction of ADAMTS-1 is drastically reduced in rats when the preovulatory synthesis of progesterone is inhibited with epostane (Espey et al. 2000b) or in mice that are null for PR (Robker et al. 2000). The temporal pattern of these events indicates that ADAMTS-1 is a target of PR and acts downstream to mediate some aspect of PR-regulated ovarian activity that culminates in the rupture of a follicle. The pattern of expression of cathepsin L is more complex but appears to be responsive to PR in the ovulating follicle. Whether or not PR acts directly or indirectly to control the expression of these two distinct proteases remains to be determined. To date no consensus PR response element (PRRE) has been identified in the ADAMTS-1 promoter and evidence for a direct effect of PR has not been observed in culture. Therefore, we propose at the moment that PR controls the expression of an intermediary step that may be a specific signaling pathway that impacts transcription factor activity at the promoter.

ADAMTS-1 is a modular protein with several putative functional domains. It needs to be determined which domains, if any, specifically impact ovulation. Three major sites of action are likely. That ADAMTS-1 is a potent protease has been determined by its ability to activate the bait region of α2-macroglobulin (Kuno et al. 1999). As an active secreted protease, it is likely to initiate one or more proteolytic cascades that account for the observed phenotype of the mice null for PR. ADAMTS-1-like ADAMTS-4 (also expressed in the ovary) may also control the amount and the cellular location of various proteoglycans. Brevican and versican are present in follicular fluid, perlican is present in the thecal cell compartment. The cell-surface proteoglycans such as syndecan or glypican may be on either granulosa cells or theca cells (Ishiguro et al. 1999; MacArthur et al. 2000). Both ADAMTS-1 and ADAMTS-4 have been shown to degrade aggrecan and brevican (Kuno et al. 2000; Nakamura et al. 2000; Tortorella et al. 2000). Therefore, it is highly likely that the proteoglycans present in ovarian follicles are targets of ADAMTS-1 action. By altering the local concentrations of proteoglycans, ADAMTS-1 could also regulate the activity of specific growth factors, such as GDF-9, FGF-2 and FGF-7, EGF, TGF-α, or Wnts whose activity is known to be blocked/modified by proteoglycans (Park et al. 2000). In the absence of ADAMTS-1, the activation of one or more of these potent growth factors in the follicular fluid would be prevented.

The function for ADAMTS-1 in the follicle may be mediated by its ability to interact with specific cellular signaling molecules through disintegrin or thrombospondin motifs at the carboxy terminus of the protein (Kuno et al. 1999). Like some other ADAM proteins, ADAMTS-1 may be a signaling protein that regulates some aspect of granulosa cell function via interactions with specific cell surface G-protein coupled receptors (GPCRs), integrins, and tetraspan proteins (Woods and Couchman 2000; Yauch et al. 2000). ADAMTS-1, like thrombospondin 1 (TS-1), is also a potent anti-angiogenic factor that may interact with integrins (Vazquez et al. 1999). Although TS-1 and -2 are expressed in ovarian follicles (Bagavandoss et al. 1998), the specific roles of thrombospondins and ADAMTS-1 have not yet been clearly delineated. Based on our limited understanding of ADAMTS-1 in mammalian cells, it is difficult to predict which of its multiple functions might be critical for impacting the process of ovulation. Mutations of ADAMTS-1, ADAMTS-4, and ADAMTS-9 genes are clearly needed to resolve this important area of ovarian cell function and ovulation.

Cathepsin L is another LH- and PR-regulated gene in the ovary that was identified by cDNA array technology (Robker et al. 2000). Cathepsin L is a member of the papain family of enzymes. It is commonly a lysosomal protease, but it is also secreted from certain endocrine cells such as Sertoli cells of the testis and placental trophoblasts and from certain tumors (Ishidoh and Kominami 1998). In the cat uterus, cathepsin L is also regulated by progesterone (Jaffe et al. 1989). The function of cathepsin L in the ovary appears to be complex. This enzyme is expressed in granulosa cells of follicles at several different stages of development in response to both FSH and LH. In addition, its expression in ovulatory follicles is impaired in PR-null mice (Robker et al. 2000). A functional link between PR-regulated expression of ADAMTS-1 and cathepsin L is not immediately obvious, but this issue will be clarified as more information is gained about the specific roles of these proteases in the ovulation process. Cathepsin L, like cathepsin G, may activate protease-activated receptors, PARs (Sambrano et al. 2000).

PACAP and the type-I PACAP receptor (PAC1) are also LH-inducible genes that have been shown to be responsive to regulation by progesterone and PR-antagonists in vivo and in vitro (Gras et al. 1999; Ko et al. 1999; Ko and Park-Sarge 2000; Park et al. 2000). However, expression of PACAP is not altered in mice null for PR (K.H. Doyle and J.S. Richards, unpublished observations). Therefore, these results indicate that PR is not essential for PACAP but may regulate other cell signaling events during process of ovulation in mice.

4.5 Regulated Expression of Wnts and Frizzleds in the Ovary

Other factors that have been shown to impact ovarian cell function and follicular organization are members of the Wnt and Frizzled family of signaling molecules. Wnts are secreted, extracellular signaling molecules that act locally to control diverse developmental processes such as cell fate specification, cell proliferation, and cell differentiation (Cadigan and Nusse 1997; Miller et al. 1999). Wnts transduce their signals by binding to G-protein coupled receptors of the Frizzled family to activate distinct signaling cascades (Slusarski et al. 1997; Lin and Perrimon 1999; Liu et al. 2001). In the canonical pathway, Wnts/Frizzleds act to hyperphosphorylate disheveled (Dv)1 (Mao et al. 2001), a cytoplasmic scaffolding protein and glycogen synthase kinase 3β (GSK-3β) leading to the release of β-catenin. Soluble β-catenin heterodimerizes with members of the T cell factor/lymphoid enhancer factor (Tcf/Lef) family of transcription factors to regulate expression of selected target genes such as c-myc (He et al. 1998). Some Wnts activate Frizzled receptors that signal via intracellular calcium, protein kinase C and/or calmodulin-dependent kinases (Kuhl et al. 2000). The Wnt/Frizzled signaling pathways are further modulated by co-receptors (proteoglycans and/or arrow/LRP-5/LRP-6) (Lin and Perrimon 1999; Tsuda et al. 1999; Alexander et al. 2000; Pinson et al. 2000; Tamai et al. 2000; Wehrli et al. 2000; Mao et al. 2001) and by antagonists such as the secreted frizzled-related proteins (sFRPs; Rattner et al. 1997).

The Wnt/Frizzled cellular signaling pathways impact the development of reproductive organs. For example, Wnt-4 is essential for side-branching in the mammary gland, a process that likely involves regulation of BMP or FGF signaling molecules (Coleman-Krnacik and Rosen 1994; Weber-Hall et al. 1994; Phippard et al. 1996; Brisken et al. 2000; Wakefield et al. 2001). In mammary tissue, Wnt-4 is co-localized with progesterone receptor (PR), and is a target of PR action (Brisken et al. 2000). In the kidney Wnt-4 is a mesenchymal signal essential for epithelial cell differentiation (Kispert et al. 1998). Furthermore, in this tissue, Wnt-4 can be replaced by Wnt-1, Wnt-3a, Wnt-7a, or Wnt-7b, indicating redundant or overlapping pathways with specific Frizzled receptors (Kispert et al. 1998). In pituitary gland development, Wnt-5a and BMP-4 play critical roles in cell fate, whereas Wnt-4 is important for expansion of ventral pituitary cell phenotypes. Wnt-7a-deficient mice are infertile due to abnormal development of the oviduct and uterus (Parr and McMahon 1998). Mutations of Wnt-2 and Frizzled-5 were shown to impact placental angiogenesis (Monkley et al. 1996; Ishikawa et al. 2001).

Wnt-4 is also essential for the embryonic development of the ovary. Female mice null for Wnt-4 have sex-reversed ovaries that at birth are depleted of oocytes and contain supporting cells expressing genes characteristic of testis development such as Müllerian inhibiting substance (MIS) (Vainio et al. 1999). Since mice null for Wnt-4 die at birth, we have analyzed by RT-PCR and in situ hybridization the expression of Wnt-4 in the adult ovary. Our results show that Wnt-4 is expressed in granulosa cells of small primary follicles containing one or two layers of cells and in granulosa cells of preovulatory follicles (Hsieh et al. 2002). Wnt-4 expression is increased in granulosa cells by the LH surge and reaches its highest level in corpora lutea. Unlike the mammary gland, Wnt-4 is not a target of PR in the ovary (Hsieh et al. 2002), perhaps because PRA rather than PRB plays a primary role in the follicle (Mulac-Jericevic et al. 2000; Conneely et al. 2001). Wnt-4 may control different aspects of granulosa cell and luteal cell function depending on which Frizzled receptors are present. Although it is not yet clear which Frizzled receptor is present in primary follicles, our results show that Frizzled-1 is induced transiently by the LH surge. It is localized to granulosa cells of ovulating follicles between 4–12 h after exposure to the LH surge, just prior to ovulation. Thus, Frizzled-1 may control the expression of genes (ADAMTS-1 or cathepsin L?) that impact the ovulation process. In contrast, Frizzled-4 is preferentially expressed at elevated levels in corpora lutea (Richards 2001; Hsieh et al. 2002;

Richards et al. 2002b). Thus, Frizzled-4 may be a receptor for Wnt-4 in this tissue. Mice null for Frizzled-4 also exhibit reproductive (ovarian?) defects, but the exact nature of this is not yet known (J. Nathans, personal communication).

4.6 Summary

The multiplicity of genes regulated by the actions of LH in specific granulosa cell and cumulus cell microenvironments of the follicle during ovulation has now revealed how complex and finely tuned the ovulation process is. Although many proteases are expressed in the ovary and are hormonally regulated, the novel proteases ADAMTS-1 and cathepsin L, rather than the MMPs, have gained particular recognition. These may play critical roles in the eventual rupture of the follicle at the ovarian surface. Rupture is only one part of ovulation. Another important aspect is the actual release of the oocyte from the ovulation pore. Several recent studies have shown that the production of the matrix that is evidenced by cumulus expansion is somehow critical for extrusion to occur and for the oocyte to travel into the oviduct. At any point the oocyte may be trapped within a non-ovulating structure. Lastly, if the events of ovulation fail to occur before the events of luteinization are complete, oocytes are destined to degenerate within the non-ovulating structures.

Acknowledgements. Supported in part by NIH-HD-16272, HD-16229, and a Specialized Cooperative Centers Program in Reproductive Research (SCCPRR)-HD-07495.

References

Alexander CM, Reichman F, Hinkes MT, Lincecum J, Becker KA, Cumberledge S, Bernfield M (2000) Syndecan-1 is required for Wnt-1-induced mammary tumorigenesis in mice. Nat Genet 25:329–332

Bagavandoss P, Sage EH, Vernon RB (1998) Secreted protein, acidic and rich in cysteine (SPARC) and thrombospondin in the developing follicle and corpus luteum of the rat. J Histochem Cytochem 46:1043–1049

Brisken C, Heineman A, Chavarria T, Elenbaas B, Tan J, Dey SK, McMahon JA, McMahon AP, Weinberg RA (2000) Essential function of Wnt-4 in mammary gland development downstream of progesterone signaling. Genes Dev 14:650–654

Cadigan KM, Nusse R (1997) Wnt signaling: a common theme in animal development. Genes Dev 11:3286–3305

Chen L, Zhang H, Powers RW, Russell PT, Larsen WJ (1996) Covalent linkage between proteins of the inter-alpha-inhibitor family and hyaluronic acid is mediated by a factor produced by granulosa cells. J Biol Chem 271:19409–19414

Clemens JW, Kraus WL, Katenellenbogen BS, Richards JS (1998) Hormone induction of progesterone receptor (PR) mRNA and activation of PR promoter regions in ovarian granulosa cells: evidence for a role of cAMP but not estradiol. Mol Endocrinol 12:1201–1214

Coleman-Krnacik S, Rosen JM (1994) Differential temporal and spatial gene expression of fibroblast growth factor family members during mouse mammary gland development. Mol Endocrinol 8:218–229

Conneely OM, Mulac-Jericevic B, Lydon JP, DeMayo FJ (2001) Reproductive functions of the progesterone receptor isoforms: lessons from knockout mice. Mol Cell Endocrinol 179:97–103

Couse JF, Korach KS (1999) Estrogen receptor null mice: what have we learned and where will they lead us? Endocrine Rev 20:358–417

Couse JF, Bunch DO, Lindzey J, Schomberg DW, Korach KS (1999) Prevention of the polycystic ovarian phenotype and characterization of ovulatory capacity in the estrogen receptor-α knockout mouse. Endocrinology 140:5855–5894

Curry TE, Osteen KG (2001) Cyclic changes in the matrix metalloproteinase system in the ovary and uterus. Biol Reprod 64:1285–1296

Davis BJ, Lennard DE, Lee CA, Tiano HF, Morham SG, Wetsel WC, Langenbach R (1999) Anovulation in cyclo-oxygenase-2-deficient mice is restored by prostaglandin E2 and interleukin-1β. Endocrinology 140:2685–2696

Dinchuk JE, Car BD, Focht RJ, Johnston JJ, Jaffee BD, Covington MB, Contel NR, Eng VM, Collins RJ, Czerniak PM, Gorry SA, Trzaskos J (1995) Renal abnormalities and an altered inflammatory response in mice lacking cyclooxygenase II. Nature 378:406–409

Elvin JA, Clark AT, Wang P, Wolfman NM, Matzuk MM (1999) Paracrine actions of growth differentiation factor-9 in the mammalian ovary. Mol Endocrinol 13:1035–1048

Eppig JJ (1979) FSH stimulates hyaluronic acid synthesis by oocyte-cumulus cell complexes from mouse preovulatory follicles. Nature 281:483–484

Eppig JJ (1991) Intercommunication between the mammalian oocytes and companion somatic cells. Bioessays 13:569–574

Espey LL, Ujoka T, Russell DL, Skelsey M, Vladu B, Robker RL, Okamura H, Richards JS (2000a) Induction of early growth response protein-1 (Egr-1) gene expression in the rat ovary in response to an ovulatory dose of hCG. Endocrinology 141:2385–2391

Espey LL, Yoshioka S, Russell DL, Robker RL, Fujii S, Richards JS (2000b) Ovarian expression of a disintegrin metalloproteinase with thrombospondin motifs during ovulation in the gonadotropin-primed immature rat. Biol Reprod 62:1090–1095

Fulop C, Kamath RV, Li Y, Otto JM, Salustri A, Olsen BR, Glant TT, Hascall VC (1997) Coding sequence, exon-intron structure and chromosomal localization of murine TNF-stimulated gene 6 that is specifically expressed by expanding cumulus cell-oocyte complexes. Gene 202:95–102

Gras S, Hannibal J, Fahrenkrug J (1999) Pituitary adenylate cyclase-activating polypeptide is an auto/paracrine stimulator of acute progesterone accumulation and subsequent luteinization in cultured periovulatory granulosa/lutein cells. Endocrinology 140:2199–2205

He TC, Sparks AB, Rago C, Hermeking H, Zawel L, da Costa LT, Morin PJ, Vogelstein B, Kinzler KW (1998) Identification of c-MYC as a target of the APC pathway. Science 281:1509–1512

Hess KA, Chen L, Larsen WJ (1999) Inter-α-inhibitor binding to hyaluronan in the cumulus extracellular matrix is required for optimal ovulation and development of mouse oocytes. Biol Reprod 61:436–443

Hizaki H, Segi E, Sugimoto Y, Hirose M, Saji T, Ushikubi F, Matsuoka T, Noda Y, Tanaka T, Yoshida N, Narumiya S, Ichikawa A (1999) Abortive expansion of the cumulus and impaired fertility in mice lacking the prostaglandin E receptor subtype EP2. Proc Natl Acad Sci USA 96:10501–10506

Hsieh M, Johnson M, Greenberg NM, Richards JS (2002) Regulated expression of Wnt and Frizzled Signals in the rodent ovary. Endocrinology (in press)

Ishidoh K, Kominami E (1998) Gene regulation and extracellular functions of procathepsin L. J Biol Chem 379:131–135

Ishiguro K, Kojima T, Taguchi O, Saito H, Muramatsu T, Kadomatsu K (1999) Syndecan-4 expression is associated with follicular atresia in mouse ovary. Histchem Cell Biol 112:25–33

Ishikawa T, Tamai Y, Zorn AM (2001) Mouse Wnt receptor Frd5 is essential for yolk sac and placental angiogenesis. Development 128:25–33

Jaffe RC, Donnelly KM, Mavrogianis PA, Verhage HG (1989) Molecular cloning and characterization of a progesterone-dependent cat endometrial secretory protein complementary deoxyribonucleic acid. Mol Endocrinol 3:1807–1814

Joyce IM, Pendola FL, O'Brien M, Eppig JJ (2001) Regulation of prostaglandin-endoperoxide synthase 2 messenger ribonucleic acid expression in mouse granulosa cells during ovulation. Endocrinology 142:3187–3197

Kispert A, Vanio S, McMahon AP (1998) Wnt-4 is a mesenchymal signal for epithelial transformation of metanephric mesenchyme in the developing kidney. Development 125:4225–4234

Ko C, Park-Sarge OK (2000) Progesterone receptor activation mediates LH-induced type-I pituitary adenylate cyclase activating polypeptide receptor (PAC(1)) gene expression in rat granulosa cells. Biochem Biophys Res Commun 277:270–279

Ko C, In YH, Park-Sarge OK (1999) Role of progesterone receptor activation in pituitary adenylate-cyclase activating polypeptide gene expression in rat ovary. Endocrinology 140:5185–5194

Kuhl M, Sheldahl LC, Park M, Miller JR, Moon RT (2000) The Wnt/Ca2+ pathway: a new vertebrate Wnt signaling pathway takes shape. Trends Genet 16:279–283

Kuno K, Terashima Y, Matsushima K (1999) ADAMTS-1 is an active metalloproteinase with the extracellular matrix. J Biol Chem 274:18821–18826

Kuno K, Okada Y, Kawashima H, Nakamura H, Miyasaka M, Ohno H, Matsushima K (2000) ADAMTS-1 cleaves a cartilage proteoglycan, aggrecan. FEBS Letters 478:241–245

Lee TH, Wisiewski H-G, Vilcek J (1992) A novel secretory tumor necrosis factor-inducible protein (TSG-6) is a member of the family of hyaluronate binding proteins, closely related to the adhesion receptor CD44. J Cell Biol 116:545–557

Lin X, Perrimon N (1999) Dally cooperates with Drosophila Frizzled 2 to transduce Wingless signalling. Nature 400:281–284

Liu T, DeCostanzo AJ, Liu X, Wang HY, Hallagan S, Moon RT, Malbon CC (2001) G protein signaling from activated rat Frizzled-1 to beta-catenin-Lef-Tcf pathway. Science 292:1718–1722

Lui K, Wahlberg P, Ny T (1998) Coordinated and cell-specific regulation of membrane type matrix metalloproteinase 1 (MT1-MMP) and its substrate matrix metalloproteinase 2 (MMP-2) by physiological signals during follicular development and ovulation. Endocrinology 139:4735–4738

Lydon JP, DeMayo F, Funk CR, Mani SK, Hughes AR, Montgomery CA, Shyamala G, Conneely OM, O'Malley BW (1995) Mice lacking progesterone receptor exhibit reproductive abnormalities. Genes Dev 9:2266–2278

MacArthur ME, Irving-Rodgers HF, Byers S, Rodgers RJ (2000) Identification and immunolocalization of decorin, versican, perlecan, nidogen, and chondroitin sulfate proteoglycans in bovine small-antral ovarian follicles. Biol Reprod 63:913–924

Mao J, Wang J, Liu B, Pann W, Farr GH, Flynn C, Yuan H, Takada S, Kimelman D, Li L, Wu D (2001) Low-density lipoprotein related-receptor protein-5 binds to Axin and regulates the canonical Wnt signaling pathway. Mol Cell 7:801–809

Miller JR, Hocking AM, Brown JD, Moon RT (1999) Mechanism and function of signal transduction by Wnt/beta-catenin and Wnt/Ca2+ pathways. Oncogene 18:7860–7872

Monkley SJ, Delaney SJ, Pennisi DJ, Christiansen JH, Wainwright BJ (1996) Targeted disruption of the Wnt2 gene results in placental defects. Development 122:3343–3353

Morham SG, Langenback R, Loftin CD, Tiano HF, Vouloumanos N, Jennette JC, Mahler JF, Kluckman KD, Ledford A, Lee CA, Smithies O (1995) Prostaglandin synthase 2 gene disruption causes severe renal pathology in the mouse. Cell 83:473–482

Mukhopadhyay D, Hascall VC, Day AJ, Salustri A, Fulop C (2001) Two distinct populations of tumor necrosis factor-stimulated gene-6 protein in the extracellular matrix of expanded mouse cumulus cell-oocyte complexes. Arch Biochem Biophys 394:173–181

Mulac-Jericevic B, Mullinax RA, DeMayo FJ, Lydon JP, Conneely OM (2000) Subgroup of reproductive functions of progesterone mediated by receptor-B isoform. Science 289:1751–1754

Nakamura H, Fujii Y, Inoka I, Kazuhiko S, Tanzawa K, Matsuki H, Miura R, Yamaguchi Y, Okada Y (2000) Brevican is degraded by matrix metalloproteinases and aggrecanase-1 (ADAMTS-4) at different sites. J Biol Chem 275:38885–38890

Natraj U, Richards JS (1993) Hormonal regulation, localization and functional activity of the progesterone receptor in granulosa cells of rat preovulatory follicles. Endocrinology 133:761–769

Pall M, Mikuni M, Mitsube K, Brannstrom M (2000) Time-dependent ovulation inhibition of a selective progesterone-receptor antagonist (Org 31710) and effect on ovulatory mediators in the in vitro perfused rat ovary. Biol Reprod 63:1642–1647

Park O-K, Mayo K (1991) Transient expression of progesterone receptor messenger RNA in ovarian granulosa cells after the preovulatory luteinizing hormone surge. Mol Endocrinol 5:967–978

Park J-II, Kim W-J, Wang L, Park H-J, Lee J, Park J-H, Kwon H-B, Tsafriri A, Chun S-Y (2000) Involvement of progesterone in gonadotropin-induced pituitary adenylate cyclase-activating polypeptide gene expression in preovulatory follicles of rat ovary. Mol Human Reprod 6:238–245

Park PW, Reizes O, Bernfield M (2000) Cell surface heparan sulfate proteoglycans: selective regulators of ligand-receptor encounters. J Biol Chem 275:29923–29926

Parr BZ, McMahon AP (1998) Sexually dimorphic development of the mammalian reproductive tract requires Wnt 7a. Nature 395:707–710

Phippard DJ, Weber-Hall SJ, Sharpe PT, Naylor MS, Jayatalake H, Maas R, Woo I, Roberts-Clark D, Francis-West PH, Liu YH, Maxson R, Hill RE, Dale TC (1996) Regulation of Msx-1, Msx-2, Bmp-2 and Bmp-4 during foetal and postnatal mammary gland development. Development 122:2729–2737

Pinson KI, Brennan J, Monkley S, Avery BJ, Skarnes WC (2000) An LDL-receptor-related protein mediates Wnt signaling in mice. Nature 407:535–538

Rattner A, Hsieh JC, Smallwood PM, Gilbert DJ, Copeland NG, Jenkins NA, Nathans J (1997) A family of secreted proteins contains homology to the cysteine-rich ligand binding domain of frizzled receptors. Proc Natl Acad Sci USA 94:2859–2863

Richards JS (1994) Hormonal control of gene expression in the ovary. Endocr Rev 15:725–751

Richards JS (2001) Perspective: the ovarian follicle – a perspective in 2001. Endocrinology 142:1–10

Richards JS, Russell DL, Robker RL, Dajee M, Alliston TN (1998) Molecular mechanisms of ovulation and luteinization. Mol Cell Endocrinol 145:47–54

Richards JS, Robker RL, Russell, D, Sharma CS, Espey LE, Lydon J, O'Malley BW (2000) Ovulation: a multi-gene, multi-step process. Steroids 65:559–570

Richards JS, Ochsner S, Russell DL, Falender AE, Hsieh MN, Doyle KH, Sharma Sc (2002a) Novel signaling pathways that control follicular growth and ovulation. Recent Prog Horm Res (in press)

Richards JS, Russell DL, Ochsner S, Espey LL (2002b) Ovulation: new dimensions and new regulators of the inflammatory-like response. Ann Rev Physiol 64:02.1–02.24

Robker RL, Richards JS (1998a) Hormonal control of the cell cycle in ovarian cells: proliferation versus differentiation. Biol Reprod 59:476–482

Robker RL, Richards JS (1998b) Hormone-induced proliferation and differentiation of granulosa cells: a coordinated balance of the cell cycle regulators cyclin D2 and p27KIP1. Mol Endocrinol 12:924–940

Robker RL, Russell DL, Espey LL, Lydon JP, O'Malley BW, Richards JS (2000) Progesterone-regulated genes in the ovulation process: ADAMTS-1 and cathepsin L proteases. Proc Natl Acad Sci USA 97:4689–4694

Rose UM, Hanssen RGJM, Kloosterboer HJ (1999) Development and characterization of an in vitro ovulation model using mouse ovarian follicles. Biol Reprod 61:503–511

Salustri A, Camaioni A, Di Giacomo M, Fulop C, Hascall VC (1999) Hyaluronan and proteoglycans in ovarian follicles. Hum Reprod Update 5:293–301

Sambrano GR, Huang W, Faruqi T, Mahrus S, Craik C, Coughlin SR (2000) Cathepsin G activates protease-activated receptor-4 in human platelets. J Biol Chem 275:6819–6823

Sato H, Kajikawa S, Kuroda S, Horisawa Y, Nakamura N, Kaga N, Kakinuma C, Kato K, Morishita H, Niwa H, Miyazaki J (2001) Impaired fertility in female mice lacking urinary trypsin inhibitor. Biochem Biphys Res Comm 281:1154–1160

Sharma CS, Richards JS (2000) Regulation of AP1 (Jun/Fos) factor expression and activation in ovarian granulosa cells: relation of JunD and Fra2 to terminal differentiation. J Biol Chem 275:33718–33728

Sharma SC, Richards JS (2002) Expression and functional analysis of the mouse progesterone receptor promoter-luciferase activation in granulosa cells. In preparation

Sirois J, Richards JS (1993) Transcriptional regulation of the rat prostaglandin endoperoxide synthase 2 gene in granulosa cells. J Biol Chem 268:21931–21938

Sirois J, Simmons DL, Richards JS (1992) Hormonal regulation of messenger ribonucleic acid encoding a novel isoform of prostaglandin endoperoxide H synthase in rat preovulatory follicles. J Biol Chem 267:11586–11592

Slusarski DC, Corces VG, Moon RT (1997) Interaction of Wnt and a Frizzled homologue triggers G-protein-linked phosphatidylinositol signalling. Nature 390:410–413

Tamai K, Semenov M, Kato Y, Spokony R, Liu C, Katsuyama Y, Hess F, Saint-Jeannet J-P, He X (2000) LDL-receptor-related proteins in Wnt signal transduction. Nature 407:530–535

Tilley SL, Audoly LP, Hicks EH, Kim H-S, Flannery PJ, Coffman TM, Koller BH (1999) Reproductive failure and reduced blood pressure in mice lacking the EP2 prostaglandin E2 receptor. J Clin Invest 103:1539–1545

Tortorella MD, Pratta M, Liu R-Q, Austin J, Ross OH, Abbaszade I, Burn T, Arner E (2000) Sites of aggrecan cleavage by recombinant human aggrecanase-1 (ADAMTS-4). J Biol Chem 275:18566–18573

Tsuda M, Kamimura K, Nakato H, Archer M, Staatz W, Fox B, Humphrey M, Olson S, Futch T, Kaluza V, Siegfried E, Stam L, Selleck SB (1999) The cell-surface proteoglycan Dally regulates Wingless signalling in *Drosophila*. Nature 400:276–280

Vainio S, Heikkila M, Kispert A, Chin N, McMahon AP (1999) Female development in mammals is regulated by Wnt-4 signalling. Nature 397:405–409

Vazquez F, Hastings G, Ortega M-A, Lane TF, Oikemus S, Lombardo M, Iruela-Arispe ML (1999) METH-1, a human ortholog of ADAMTS-1, and METH-2 are members of a new family of proteins with angio-inhibitory activity. J Biol Chem 274:23349–23357

Wakefield LM, Piek E, Bottinger EP (2001) TGF-beta signaling in mammary gland development and rumorigenesis. J Mammary Gland Biol Neoplasia 6:67–82

Weber-Hall SJ, Phippard DJ, Niemeyer CC, Dale TC (1994) Developmental and hormonal regulation of Wnt gene expression in the mouse mammary gland. Differentiation 57:205–214

Wehrli M, Dougan ST, Caldwell K, O'Keefe L, SchwartZ S, Vaizel-Ohayon D, Schejter E, Tomlinson A, DiNardo S (2000) *Arrow* encodes an LDL-receptor-related protein essential for Wingless signaling. Nature 407:527–530

Weigel PH, Hascall VC, Tammi M (1997) Hyaluronan synthase. J Biol Chem 272:13997–14000

Werb Z (1989) Proteinases and matrix degradation. In: Kelly WN (ed) Textbook of rheumatology. WB Saunders, Philadelphia, pp 300–321

Woods A, Couchman JR (2000) Integrin modulation by lateral association. J Biol Chem 275:24233–24236

Yauch RL, Kazarov AR, Desai B, Lee RT, Hemler ME (2000) Direct extracellular contact between integrin α3β1 and TM4SF protein CD151. J Biol Chem 275:9230–9238

Yoshioka S, Ochsner S, Russell DL, Ujioka T, Fujii S, Richards JS, Espey LL (2000) Expression of tumor necrosis factor-stimulated gene-6 in the rat ovary in response to an ovulatory dose of gonadotropin. Endocrinology 141:4114–4119

Zhou L, Yoneda M, Zhao M, Yingsung W, Yoshida N, Kitagawa Y, Kawamura K, Suzuki t, Kimata K (2001) Defect in SHAP-hyaluronan complex causes severe female infertility: a study by inaction of the bikunin gene in mice. J Biol Chem 276:7693–7696

5 Phenotypic Effects of Knockout of Oocyte-Specific Genes

S. Varani, M.M. Matzuk

5.1 Introduction 63
5.2 Knockout of Oocyte-Specific Genes 64
5.3 Identification of Additional Novel Oocyte-Specific Genes 74
References 77

5.1 Introduction

Folliculogenesis is a complex process requiring both extragonadal and intragonadal factors aimed at the production of fully mature oocytes, ready to be fertilized. The follicle is the functional unit of the ovary, where the tight communication between the oocyte and the surrounding somatic cells allows controlled growth and differentiation of the oocyte to form the ovum, the female gamete that supplies the many proteins and factors necessary for fertilization events and early embryonic development. At birth, the female has a finite oocyte population. By day 2 after birth in the mouse, a layer of squamous granulosa cells surrounds the oocytes to form quiescent primordial follicles. Unknown intragonadal factors regulate the entry of primordial follicles into the growing phase. At this point the follicle is committed to a program of growth and differentiation that culminates in either apoptotic death of the granulosa cells (atresia) and oocyte or ovulation of the mature oocyte. Initiation of follicle growth is marked by a squamous to cuboidal morphological transition of the pregranulosa cells to form a one-layer primary follicle.

As follicular growth progresses, granulosa cells proliferate, fibroblast-like cells from the interstitium are recruited to form the theca layer, and the oocyte grows and secretes an extracellular glycoprotein matrix, the zona pellucida. The final stages of follicular growth are marked by the appearance of scattered fluid-filled spaces between granulosa cells, which collapse into a single antral cavity. The antral follicles that become responsive to gonadotropins are selected for further development to form preovulatory follicles, in which a meiotically competent oocyte protrudes into the antral cavity, surrounded by cumulus granulosa cells. The luteinizing hormone (LH) surge triggers the release of the oocyte from meiotic arrest, breakdown of the follicle wall, and extrusion of the cumulus–oocyte complex into the oviduct. The oocyte completes meiosis I and progresses to the metaphase stage of meiosis II, where it arrests again until fertilization. The granulosa cells remaining in the ovary undergo luteinization and form the corpus luteum, a transient endocrine organ that produces progesterone, essential for uterine preparation and maintenance of pregnancy.

With the development of transgenic mouse technology, it is now possible to alter the expression of a selected gene and observe the effect on the development and function of a specific tissue or the entire organism. Use of the transgenic approach to study gonadogenesis and folliculogenesis in mice is expanding our understanding of mammalian ovarian development and physiology as well as generating mouse models to study human infertility.

Our laboratory has been focusing on identifying and characterizing oocyte-specific genes, with the goal of dissecting the active role of the oocyte in the regulation of folliculogenesis, ovulation, fertilization, and early embryonic development. In addition, oocyte-specific gene products may provide future tissue-specific pharmacological targets for non-hormonal contraception.

5.2 Knockout of Oocyte-Specific Genes

While there is long-standing evidence that somatic cells support oocyte growth and maturation (Eppig et al. 1997), the reciprocal phenomenon of oocytes modulating granulosa-cell and cumulus-cell functions has become clear only over the past decade. In mutant mice that lack germ

Table 1. Knockout of oocyte-specific genes

Gene/mutant mouse	Protein function/family	Knockout phenotype
Factor in the germline (*Figla*)	Helix-loop-helix transcription factor	Female infertility, absence of primordial follicles (Soyal et al. 2000)
Zona pellucida 1 (*Zp1*)	Zona pellucida 1 glycoprotein	Female subfertility, abnormal/thin zona pellucida (Rankin et al. 1999)
Zona pellucida 2 (*Zp2*)	Zona pellucida 2 glycoprotein	Female infertility, thins/abnormal zona pellucida (Rankin et al. 2001)
Zona pellucida 3 (*Zp3*)	Zona pellucida 3 glycoprotein	Female infertility, no zona pellucida (Liu et al. 1996; Rankin et al. 1996)
Growth differentiation factor 9 (*Gdf9*)	Transforming growth factor β	Female infertility, block in preantral follicle development (Dong et al. 1996)
Bone morphogenetic protein 15 (*Bmp15*)	Transforming growth factor β	Female subfertility, defects in ovulation and fertilization (Yan et al. 2001a)
Mos	Serine/threonine kinase, oncoprotein	Female subfertility, parthenogenetic activation of oocytes, ovarian teratomas (Colledge et al. 1994; Hashimoto et al. 1994)
Maternal antigen that embryos require (*Mater*)	Unknown family; contains leucine-rich and leucine zipper domains	Female infertility, block of embryonic development at two-cell stage (Tong et al. 2000)

cells, follicles do not form (Coulombre and Russell 1954), and pharmaceutical ablation of oocytes in rats results in defective folliculogenesis (Hirshfield 1994). Several genes expressed specifically by oocytes in female mice have been cloned and characterized so far. Targeted mutation of such genes has started to uncover the central role played by the oocyte during folliculogenesis and early embryonic development (see Table 1).

5.2.1 Figα Function in Primordial Follicle Development

Factor in the germline alpha (Figα or *Figla*) is an oocyte-specific basic-loop-helix transcription factor expressed in germ cells of the prenatal mouse ovary as well as primordial and growing oocytes (Liang et al. 1997). Figα was initially cloned as a transcription factor that binds with a ubiquitous partner to an upstream E box (CANNTG) in the promoter of the zona pellucida genes to regulate their expression in oocytes. Targeting of the *Figla* gene demonstrated that this factor plays an essential role in primordial follicle formation in perinatal ovaries (Soyal et al. 2000). While oocytes are present in the mutant ovary prenatally at embryonic day 18, in newborn mutant ovaries somatic cells do not adhere to and surround the oocytes. By postnatal day 1, the oocytes begin to disappear. Because granulosa cells and oocytes fail to form primordial follicles, the oocytes are irretrievably lost from the postnatal ovary and the adult females end up completely infertile. Oocytes of *Figla* mutant mice progress normally to prophase of meiosis I, ruling out the possibility of a block in meiosis as the cause of the oocyte loss. Figα may induce the expression of oocyte factors (secreted or transmembrane proteins) that in turn act on the surrounding somatic cells to recruit pregranulosa cells to form primordial follicles. These studies demonstrate how the oocyte, through the regulation of specific genes, plays a crucial role in the initial growth and development of the follicle.

5.2.2 The Function of the Zona Pellucida

An extracellular matrix surrounds all vertebrate eggs. In mammals, this matrix, known as the zona pellucida, is secreted by the oocyte, and is important for survival of growing oocytes, successful fertilization, and the passage of early embryos through the oviduct (reviewed by Rankin and Dean 2000). The zona pellucida is composed of three major glycoproteins, ZP1, ZP2, and ZP3, each encoded by a single copy gene. Oocytes that enter the growing pool begin to secrete the zona pellucida proteins which in turn form an organized extracellular matrix with ZP2 and ZP3, present in stoichiometric amounts, connected by ZP1, in less abundance than the other two zona pellicuda proteins, functioning as a bridge between the other two.

Mouse lines with targeted mutations of each of the zona pellucida genes have been generated. Mouse oocytes lacking any single zona pellucida protein continue to synthesize and secrete the other two proteins; however, the mutant mice have structural defects in their zona pellucida, associated with varying degrees of defects in folliculogenesis, fertilization, and early embryonic development (Liu et al. 1996; Rankin et al. 1996, 1999, 2001).

Female mice with a *Zp3*-null mutation are infertile (Liu et al. 1996; Rankin et al. 1996). The main defect in these mutant mice is the complete absence of a zona pellucida. Morphometric analysis of *Zp3*-null ovaries shows a marked reduction of early antral follicles compared to wild-type ovaries (Rankin et al. 2001), suggesting that the absence of the zona pellucida compromises the ability to develop antral follicles. The surviving follicles demonstrate further defects at the preovulatory stage, and a well-organized cumulus–oocyte complex fails to form. Furthermore, after hormonal stimulation, few ovulated eggs are recovered in the oviduct, and no two-cell embryos are recovered after mating superovulated mutant females with wild-type males.

Mouse lines with a targeted mutation of the *Zp1* gene have also been generated (Rankin et al. 1999). In contrast to the infertility and lack of zona matrix of *Zp3* mutant mice, *Zp1* mutant females are fertile, although their litters are half the size of wild-type mice. Although a zona pellucida is present around growing and ovulated oocytes, it is thinner than normal and structurally compromised. In a fraction of the growing oocytes, this results in ectopic localization of granulosa cells between the zona and the egg membrane. Morphometric analysis shows a decrease in the number of mid-to-late antral follicles (Rankin et al. 2001), and in those follicles that develop to the preovulatory phase, the defective matrix results in an accentuated perivitelline space, often containing cumulus granulosa cells that have undergone expansion. Despite these defects, *Zp1*-mutant females ovulate a similar number of eggs as wild-type females. The reduced litter size is most likely a consequence of loss of early embryos, as the fertilization rate of mutants is normal but the number of two-cell stage embryos is greatly reduced; this is probably due to the inability of the compromised matrix to protect the early embryos during their development in the oviduct.

Mice that lack the other zona pellucida gene, *Zp2*, have an intermediate phenotype between the other two zona pellucida-knockout mouse lines (Rankin et al. 2001). *Zp2*-null female mice are infertile; oocytes develop a thin zona pellucida early in oogenesis that is not sustained through the antral stage of folliculogenesis and is lost in ovulated eggs. Similar to *Zp1* and *Zp3* mutant mice, the early stages of folliculogenesis appear normal, with the first defects being evident in antral follicles. At this stage, the cumulus granulosa cell–oocyte complexes are highly disorganized, with loose association of germ cells with the surrounding somatic cells. Relatively few eggs are ovulated and the sterility of *Zp2* mutant females can be attributed to both the small number of zona-free eggs that reach the oviduct and the failure of fertilized eggs to develop into two-cell stage embryos.

These extensive studies demonstrate that the three zona pellucida components are necessary for the formation of a functional extracellular matrix, although only ZP3 is absolutely necessary for the zona formation. Furthermore, strong evidence supports the conclusion that disruption of a functional zona matrix effects the communication between the oocyte and surrounding granulosa cells, resulting in defects in folliculogenesis and altering the developmental potential of mutant embryos

5.2.3 Oocyte-Secreted Proteins Which Regulate Somatic Cell Functions

Several studies report evidence of factors secreted from the oocyte that influence granulosa cell proliferation and differentiation (reviewed by Eppig et al. 1997). One of these is growth differentiation factor (GDF)-9, an oocyte-specific member of the transforming growth factor (TGF)-β superfamily of secreted growth factors. *Gdf9* is first expressed by oocytes in primary follicles, and its expression persists in the oocyte through ovulation (McGrath et al. 1995; Elvin et al. 2000). We have generated knockout mice deficient in GDF-9 (Dong et al. 1996). Heterozygotes of both sexes and male homozygous for the deletion are fertile, but female homozygous mutant mice are completely infertile. Formation of the mutant ovary appears normal; primordial follicles form, are recruited to initiate follicular growth, and advance to the primary type 3b stage where the oocyte is surrounded by a single layer of granulosa cells. At this point, the oocyte degenerates, and the somatic cells undergo morphological and functional changes and form luteinized nests, corpora lutea-like structures that secrete estrogen and progesterone (Elvin et al. 1999). In addition, the mutant primary follicles present several structural and biochemical changes (Elvin et al. 1999; Carabatsos et al. 1998). Among the changes that occur in the oocyte are defects in meiotic competence, including abnormal germinal vesicle breakdown, spontaneous parthenogenetic activation, and an increased rate of growth of the oocyte. In the absence of GDF-9 the majority of the granulosa cells appear to remain dormant and fail to either proliferate or die (Elvin et al. 1999). Kit ligand, a growth factor secreted by granulosa cells signaling to the oocyte through its receptor, KIT, is upregulated in primary follicles of GDF-9-deficient ovaries (Elvin et al. 1999). This may account for the increased size of oocytes in type 3b follicles.

In wild-type ovaries, a thecal layer begins to form in type 3b follicles, when cells expressing theca cell-specific markers start to associate with the follicle and a complete ring of these theca cells forms by the multilayer preantral stage just outside the granulosa cell basement membrane. In contrast to wild-type mice, a morphologically distinct thecal layer is not detected by light and electron microscopy in GDF-9-deficient ovaries (Dong et al. 1996). Cells expressing theca cells-specific markers are scattered in the interstitium and not associated with follicles (Elvin et al. 1999).

Although GDF-9 is present at all stages of folliculogenesis, the knockout only allowed us to determine its earliest essential role in folliculogenesis. Additional studies by our group (Elvin et al. 1999) have subsequently shown that GDF-9 acts in preovulatory follicles to induce cumulus cell expansion via induction of hyaluronan synthase 2 and regulates the differential expression of other mural and cumulus granulosa cell-expressed genes. These results support the hypothesis that the gradient of oocyte-secreted factors is responsible for the different phenotypes of these two cell types. It is still unclear how GDF-9 acts at specific times during folliculogenesis, although it is present throughout the entire process. GDF-9 might be produced by the oocyte in an inactive form and require activation at specific time-points, or its receptor on somatic cells might be developmentally regulated during folliculogenesis. Uncovering the GDF-9 signaling pathway will be instrumental in understanding the biological processes that GDF-9 controls.

Bone morphogenetic protein (BMP)-15 is another oocyte-specific member of the TGF-β superfamily (Dube et al. 1998). BMP-15 importance in ovarian function was demonstrated initially in sheep, where the X-linked *BMP15* gene was shown to be mutated in *Inverdale* and *Hanna* sheep carrying the fecundity X (*FecX^I* and *FecX^H*) mutations (Galloway et al. 2000). Both strains have mutations in the mature peptide sequence. Sheep heterozygous for these mutations show increased ovulation rate resulting in more twins and triplets, while homozygous sheep are infertile, with a block in folliculogenesis that phenocopies the mouse *Gdf9* knockout. Our group has cloned the mouse and human *BMP15* genes (Dube et al. 1998) and generated *Bmp15* knockout mice (Yan et al. 2001b). Female mutant mice are fertile, although they show a reduction in litter sizes compared to wild-type mice. Histologically. the mutant ovaries are indistinguishable from wild-type and heterozygous controls. When hormonally stimulated, *Bmp15* knockout females ovulate about two thirds the number of oocytes as the controls, with some oocytes appearing to remain "trapped" in luteinized follicles in the ovary. Normally, at ovulation the cumulus granulosa cells that surround the oocyte in the ovulatory follicle accompany the oocyte into the oviduct, protecting it from enzymes at the rupture site, and remaining with the egg until after fertilization. In the *Bmp15* mutant females, a fraction of the ovulated eggs isolated in the oviduct is denuded of cumulus cells, probably because of a defect in cumulus expansion and/or interaction between the oocyte and the companion granulosa cells. Thus, although the mouse *Bmp15*-null mutation does not phenocopy the sheep mutations, it uncovers important functions of BMP15 during periovulatory events.

Given the high homology between GDF-9 and BMP-15, we determined whether there are changes of expression of BMP15 in *Gdf9* knockout ovaries and GDF-9 in *Bmp15* mutants. *Gdf9* mRNA expression was identical in *Bmp15* knockout and control ovaries. *Bmp15* mRNA levels were higher in *Gdf9* knockout ovary, a situation common in oocyte-expressed genes due to the dramatic increase in oocytes/unit volume in the *Gdf9* knockout ovaries. Therefore, the abnormalities in the *Gdf9* ovaries are not due to transcriptional inactivation of the *Bmp15* gene, nor is there a compensatory increase of *Gdf9* mRNA in *Bmp15* knockout ovaries.

To study possible genetic, physical, and functional interactions between these two factors, we intercrossed mice carrying the *Gdf9*-null mutation with *Bmp15*-null mutants. Double homozygous mutant mice show an ovarian phenotype identical to the *Gdf9*, with a block in folliculogenesis at the primary follicle stage. Interestingly, female mice homozygous for the *Bmp15* mutation and heterozygous for the *Gdf9* mutation (*Bmp15*$^{-/-}$*Gdf9*$^{+/-}$) have a more dramatic phenotype than *Bmp15* mutants. The average litter size, as well as the number of litters per month, is decreased compared to absence of *Bmp15* alone. Histological analysis of *Bmp15*$^{-/-}$*Gdf9*$^{+/-}$ ovaries shows normal folliculogenesis in a minority of cases, while most of the ovaries analyzed show abnormalities including decreased numbers of late-stage follicles, increased oocyte loss and accumulation of zona pellucida remnants in the interstitium (similar to the *Gdf9* knockout ovary), follicles with multiple oocytes, and lack of corpora lutea. Upon superovulation, the number of oocytes recovered in the oviduct of *Bmp15*$^{-/-}$*Gdf9*$^{+/-}$ females is similar to controls, but only a small percentage of the ovulated eggs can be successfully fertilized in vivo. Furthermore, all of the ovulated eggs are denuded of cumulus cells, in contrast to the *Bmp15* mutation, where only a fraction demonstrated defects in oocyte–cumulus cell adhesion. These studies have uncovered important genetic interactions between these two related oocyte-expressed factors. Furthermore, the roles of GDF-9 in periovulatory events and cumulus cell–oocyte interaction have been confirmed in vivo. Several questions remain unanswered. Is the role of GDF-9 in early folliculogenesis conserved between species? Do GDF-9 and BMP-15 utilize the same signaling pathway in the ovary? Do GDF-9 and BMP-15 have parallel complementary functions in the ovary or is one a functional antagonist of the other? Based on in vivo and in vitro findings, a model for the differential functions of these two factors in the mammalian ovary has been proposed: in mice, GDF-9 homodimers are the major signaling protein, whereas BMP-15 homodimers and BMP-15/GFD-9 heterodimers have synergistic roles. In sheep, BMP-15 homodimers seem to play a major role, although this does not rule out significant roles of BMP-15/GDF-9 heterodimers since GDF-9 mutations have not been detected and linked to ovarian phenotypes in sheep. Although these models imply that the ligands signal through a single receptor, the existence of two or more receptors cannot be ruled out. Isolation of additional proteins involved in this signaling pathway and receptor-binding studies will clarify the active forms of these ligands in mice and other species.

5.2.4 A Role for MOS in Oogenesis

One of the unique features of germ cells is their ability to form haploid gametes. This occurs through the coordination of meiosis and mitosis. The meiotic cell cycles are characterized by two consecutive M phases, meiosis I and II, without an intervening S phase, resulting in the production of haploid gametes that recover full ploidy upon fertilization. While male germ cells go through the entire program of meiotic divisions, this process is characterized by a series of starts and stops in the oocyte. The progression of meiosis is arrested at prophase I throughout the growth of the oocyte. It resumes upon the LH surge, continues to metaphase II, where it halts until fertilization occurs. The arrest at metaphase II is mediated by a cytostatic factor in which MOS, the c-mos protooncogene product, is an essential component. MOS, a cytoplasmic serine/threonine kinase, has been identified as a key regulator of meiosis in vertebrates (Sagata 1996) and invertebrates (Tachibana et al. 2000). Biochemically, MOS functions as a mitogen-activated protein kinase that phosphorylates and activates MEK (an extracellular signal-activated kinase) that in turn phosphorylates and activates mitogen-activated protein (MAP) kinase (Nebreda and Hunt 1993; Posada et al. 1993; Sagata 1997). MOS expression and function is restricted to oocytes that arrest at metaphase of meiosis II (Sagata 1996). Microinjection of *Mos* antisense oligonucleotides in mouse oocytes first proved that absence of this factor results in parthenogenetic activation and cleavage of the eggs (O'Keefe et al. 1989; Gebauer et al. 1994). These results have been confirmed with a transgenic approach (Colledge et al. 1994; Hashimoto et al. 1994). MOS deficiency in female mice results in decreased fertility due to parthenogenetic activation of ovulated oocytes, which renders them incapable of being fertilized. The small number of offspring that arise from MOS-deficient females are presumably derived from fertilization of eggs shortly after maturation and before parthenogenetic activation occurs. Furthermore, MOS-deficient female mice are subject to frequent development of teratomas, tumors composed of multiple cell types that normally derive from activation of germ cells. The oocytes develop as preimplantation-like embryos until they reach a stage comparable to 6- or 7-day embryos, after which they become disorganized and form a teratoma (Hirao and Eppig 1997). On the basis of these experiments, it has been proposed that the biological function of MOS is to prevent undesirable DNA replication or parthenogenetic activation before fertilization. However, it is still unclear how the meiotic and the embryonic mitotic cycles are coordinated by MOS.

5.2.5 MATER Is Required in Early Embryonic Development

Maternal effect genes produce mRNA or proteins that accumulate in the egg during oogenesis and control the developmental program prior to embryonic genome activation. In mice, embryonic transcription is first detected in the late one-cell zygote and is required for development beyond the two-cell stage (Flach et al. 1982). The factors governing the transition from the maternal to the embryonic genome are largely unknown.

Mater (Maternal antigen that embryos require) is a single-copy gene expressed exclusively in oocytes in the mouse (Tong and Nelson 1999). *Mater* transcripts are detected in the oocyte throughout oogenesis but are absent in early embryos, while its protein product is present through the late blastocyst stage. MATER contains a leucine-rich domain and a short leucine-zipper domain believed to be important for protein–protein interaction. *Mater*-null female mice present no phenotypic abnormalities but are completely infertile (Tong et al. 2000). MATER-deficient eggs are fertilized normally in vivo; the zygotes develop normally to the two-cell stage, but while wild-type embryos continue to divide and develop to form a multicellular organism, embryos derived from MATER-deficient eggs remain at the two-cell stage and eventually degenerate. De novo transcription occurs in the embryos lacking MATER, although it is greatly reduced, and degradation of maternal RNAs takes place. These studies show that MATER is required for embryonic development beyond the two-cell stage in mice, possibly participating in activation of the embryonic genome. Although the reduced transcription levels in the mutant embryos might account for the defect, the mechanism through which MATER and possibly other maternal effect genes control the transition from maternal to embryonic genome activation is unknown.

5.3 Identification of Additional Novel Oocyte-Specific Genes

During the past few years, we have undertaken several strategies to identify novel oocyte-specific genes. Various initial screenings lead to isolation of cDNA clones whose sequences either do not match sequences in the public databases (i.e., they are novel) or match only sequences from oocyte-derived libraries. The expression pattern of these clones was tested by multiple-tissue Northern blot analysis. The clones that showed ovary-specific expression were selected, and full-length cDNA was isolated by ovary cDNA library screening and 5′ and 3′ RACE-PCR. Their expression pattern in the ovary was then assessed by in situ RNA hybridization, and public database searches helped identifying common domains in the putative aminoacidic sequences. Several clones were pursued further: the genomic organization of the genes was identified in order to build targeting vectors, and polyclonal antibodies were raised to determine the protein expression in the ovary and for subsequent functional analyses (Fig. 1).

The first of the strategies we developed takes advantage of the high number of oocytes/volume of tissue in *Gdf9* knockout ovaries. We generated a subtractive hybridization library enriched in sequences from the ovaries of *Gdf9* knockout mice compared to ovaries from wild-type mice. Initial sequence analysis of 331 inserts from this library resulted in 31 clones that failed to match sequences in public databases; 3 of these clones were subjected to further studies and identified as oocyte-specific genes. We are currently generating knockout mice to determine the essential function of these genes in ovarian physiology.

A similar approach involves a cDNA library from germinal vesicle-stage oocytes. About 300 inserts isolated from this library were arrayed and hybridized with either radiolabeled liver or ovary cDNA. Clones that were hybridized exclusively by the ovary cDNA were sequenced and their expression pattern analyzed. The full-length cDNA of one such clone encodes an oocyte-secreted protein, OOSP1 (C. Yan et al. 2001a). Protein analysis tools indicate that OOSP1 is a secreted glycoprotein with a 21 amino acid signal peptide sequence, 5 putative N-glycosylation sites, and 3 putative disulfide bonds. OOSP1 shares about 30% amino acid identity with the placenta-specific protein 1 (PLAC1), a placental- and ectoplacental-secreted protein (Cocchia et al. 2000). Ongoing studies include the generation of recombinant OOSP1 that will be

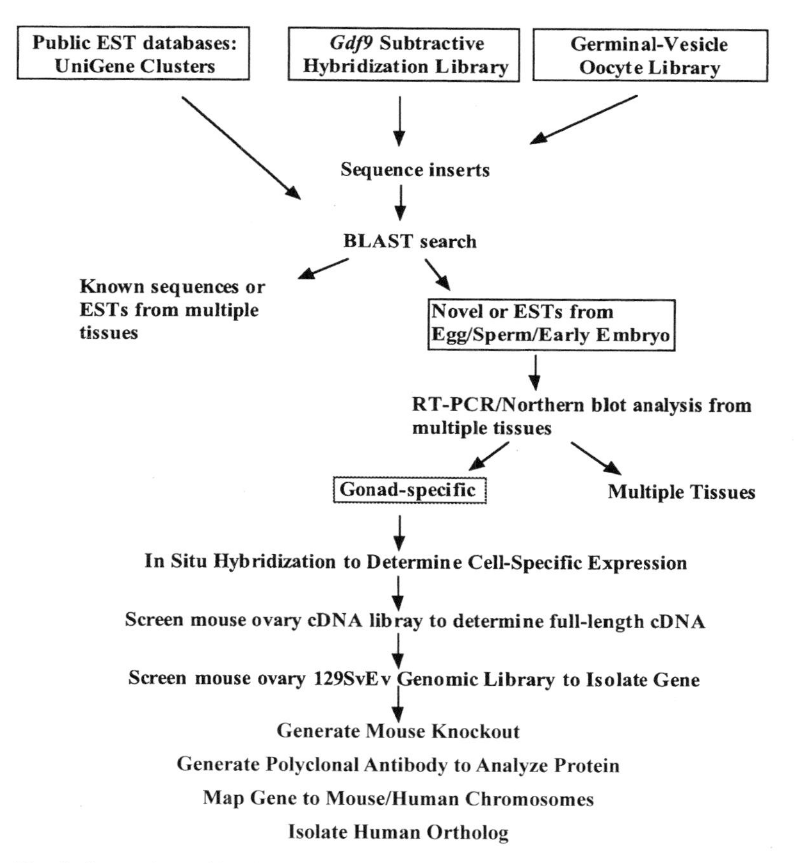

Fig. 1. Strategies to identify novel genes expressed preferentially in germ cells

tested in in vitro ovarian cultures and generation of targeted mice to define OOSP1 essential functions in ovarian physiology.

Lastly, we have also taken advantage of the enormous amount of data publicly available in the databases to identify transcripts expressed preferentially in oocytes. With an in silico subtraction strategy we downloaded several thousands publicly available expressed sequence tags (ESTs) from unfertilized egg and newborn ovary libraries and subtracted from these the ones found in libraries from other tissues

(Rajkovic et al. 2001). We identified 258 ESTs that were found in unfertilized egg libraries but not in adult mouse tissues or post-blastocyst embryo cDNA libraries. After testing the pattern of expression, three ESTs were localized exclusively to mouse oocytes in female mice. One of these encodes a 287 amino acid testis and oocyte-expressed protein which we call Ret finger protein 4 (RFPL4; Rajkovic et al. 2002). Functional domains in this protein include a RING finger domain and a B30.2 domain of unknown function, also found in other RING finger-containing proteins. Electronic protein analysis tools fail to detect a nuclear localization signal and predict that RFPL4 is localized to germ cell cytoplasm. The majority of RING finger proteins have been shown to function as E3 ubiquitin–protein ligases (Joazeiro and Weissman 2000) which transfer ubiquitin polymers from ubiquitin-conjugating enzymes to recipient proteins that are thus marked for proteolysis. Likewise, RFPL4 might function in germ cells in the targeted degradation of specific proteins. Studies aimed at identifying RFPL4 targets in germ cells and the generation of knockout mice are underway.

A second, very interesting EST, isolated from a mouse newborn ovary library, encodes a protein expressed at high levels in the ovary and weakly in testis, which we call NOBOX (newborn ovary homeobox-containing protein) (Suzumori et al. 2002). In the ovary, the *Nobox* mRNA is expressed specifically by oocytes in primordial and growing follicles. The putative protein contains a homeobox domain, a nuclear localization signal that is conserved among most homeobox proteins, and a possible site for binding to a Src homology 3 (SH3) domain. Interestingly, NOBOX is one of the first homeodomain genes preferentially expressed at early stages of mammalian folliculogenesis. Generation and characterization of *Nobox* knockout mice may give new insight into the early stages of folliculogenesis, as very little is known about the mechanisms for recruitment of primordial follicles into the growing pool in mammals.

In conclusion, mouse transgenic models are proving extremely useful in the study of mammalian oogenesis, folliculogenesis, and early embryogenesis.

Acknowledgements. Supported by NIH Grants HD33438 and HD07495.

References

Carabatsos MJ, Elvin JA, Matzuk MM, Albertini DF (1998) Characterization of oocyte and follicle development in growth differentiation factor-9-deficient mice. Dev Biol 203:373–384

Cocchia M, Huber R, Pantano S, Chen EY, Ma P, Forabosco A, Ko MS, Schlessinger D (2000) PLAC1, an Xq26 gene with a placenta-specific expression. Genomics 68:305–312

Colledge WH, Carlton MB, Udy GB, Evans MJ (1994) Disruption of c-mos causes parthenogenetic development of unfertilized mouse eggs. Nature 370:65–68

Coulombre JL, Russell ES (1954) Analysis of pleiotropism of the W-locus in the mouse: the effects of W and W^V substitution upon postnatal development of germ cells. J Exp Zool 126:277–296

Dong J, Albertini DF, Nishimori K, Kumar TR, Lu N, Matzuk MM (1996) Growth differentiation factor-9 is required during early ovarian folliculogenesis. Nature 383:531–535

Dube JL, Wang P, Elvin J, Lyons KM, Celeste AJ, Matzuk MM (1998) The bone morphogenetic protein 15 gene is X-linked and expressed in oocytes. Mol Endocrinol 12:1809–1817

Elvin JA, Clark AT, Wang P, Wolfman NM, Matzuk MM (1999) Paracrine actions of growth differentiation factor-9 in the mammalian ovary. Mol Endocrinol 13:1035–1048

Elvin JA, Yan C, Matzuk MM (2000) Oocyte-expressed TGF-beta superfamily members in female fertility. Mol Cell Endocrinol 159:1–5

Elvin JA, Yan C, Wang P, Nishimori K, Matzuk MM (1999) Molecular characterization of the follicle defects in the growth differentiation factor-9-deficient ovary. Mol Endocrinol 13:1018–1034

Eppig JJ, Chesnel F, Hirao Y, O'Brien MJ, Pendola FL, Watanabe S, Wigglesworth K (1997) Oocyte control of granulosa cell development: how and why. Hum Reprod 12:127–132

Flach G JM, Braude PR, Taylor RA, Bolton VN (1982) The transition from maternal to embryonic control in the 2-cell mouse embryo. EMBO J 1:681–686

Galloway SM, McNatty KP, Cambridge LM, Laitinen MP, Juengel JL, Jokiranta TS, McLaren RJ, Luiro K, Dodds KG, Montgomery GW, Beattie AE, Davis GH, Ritvos O (2000) Mutations in an oocyte-derived growth factor gene (BMP15) cause increased ovulation rate and infertility in a dosage-sensitive manner. Nat Genet 25:279–283

Gebauer F, Xu W, Cooper GM, Richter JD (1994) Translational control by cytoplasmic polyadenylation of c-mos mRNA is necessary for oocyte maturation in the mouse. EMBO J 13:5712–5720

Hashimoto N, Watanabe N, Furuta Y, Tamemoto H, Sagata N, Yokoyama M, Okazaki K, Nagayoshi M, Takeda N, Ikawa Y, Aizawa S (1994) Parthenogenetic activation of oocytes in c-mos-deficient mice. Nature 370:68–71

Hirao Y, Eppig JJ (1997) Parthenogenetic development of Mos-deficient mouse oocytes. Mol Rep Dev 48:391–396

Hirshfield AN (1994) Relationship between the supply of primordial follicles and the onset of follicular growth in rats. Biol Reprod 50:421–428

Joazeiro CA, Weissman AM (2000) RING finger proteins: mediators of ubiquitin ligase activity. Cell 102:549–52

Liang L-F, Soyal S, Dean J (1997) FIGalpha, a germ cell specific transcription factor involved in the coordinate expression of the zona pellucida genes. Development 124:4939–4947

Liu C, Litscher ES, Mortillo S, Sakai Y, Kinloch RA, Stewart CL, Wassarman PM (1996) Targeted disruption of the mZP3 gene results in production of eggs lacking a zona pellucida and infertility in male mice. Proc Natl Acad Sci USA 93:5431–5436

McGrath SA, Esquela AF, Lee S-J (1995) Oocyte-specific expression of growth/differentiation factor-9. Mol Endocrinol 9:131–136

Nebreda AR, Hunt T (1993) The c-mos proto-oncogene protein kinase turns on and maintains the activity of MAP kinase, but not MPF, in cell-free extracts of Xenopus oocytes and eggs. EMBO J 12:1979–1986

O'Keefe SJ, Wolfes H, Kiessling AA, Cooper GM (1989) Microinjection of antisense c-mos oligonucleotides prevents meiosis II in the maturing mouse egg. Proc Natl Acad Sci USA 86:7038–7042

Posada J, Yew N, Ahn NG, Vande Woude GF, Cooper JA (1993) Mos stimulates MAP kinase in Xenopus oocytes and activates a MAP kinase kinase in vitro. Mol Cell Biol 13:2546–53

Rajkovic A, Yan C, Klysik M, Matzuk MM (2001) Discovery of germ cell-specific transcripts by expressed sequence tag database analysis. Sterility and Fertility 76:550–554

Rajkovic A, Lee JH, Yan C, Matzuk MM (2002) The Ret Finger Protein-Like 4 gene, *Rfpl4,* encodes a putative E3 ubiquitin-protein ligase expressed in adult germ cells. Mechansims of Development 187:5–9

Rankin T, Dean J (2000) The zona pellucida: using molecular genetics to study the mammalian egg coat. Rev Reprod 5:114–121

Rankin T, Familari M, Lee E, Ginsberg A, Dwyer N, Blanchette-Mackie J, Drago J, Westphal H, Dean J (1996) Mice homozygous for an insertional mutation in the Zp3 gene lack a zona pellucida and are infertile. Development 122:2903–2910

Rankin T, Talbot P, Lee E, Dean J (1999) Abnormal zonae pellucidae in mice lacking ZP1 result in early embryonic loss. Development 126:3847–3855

Rankin TL, O'Brien M, Lee E, Wigglesworth K, Eppig J, Dean J (2001) Defective zonae pellucidae in Zp2-null mice disrupt folliculogenesis, fertility and development. Development 128:1119–1126

Sagata N (1996) Meiotic metaphase arrest in animal oocytes: its mechanisms and biological significance. Trends Cell Biol 6:22–28

Sagata N (1997) What does Mos do in oocyte and somatic cells? BioEssays 19:13–21

Soyal SM, Amleh A, Dean J (2000) FIGalpha, a germ cell-specific transcription factor required for ovarian follicle formation. Development 127:4645–4654

Suzumori S, Yan C, Matzuk MM, Rajkovic A (2002) *Nobox* is a homeobox-containing gene preferentially expressed in primordial and growing oocytes. Mechansims of Development 111:137–141

Tachibana K, Tanaka D, Isobe T, Kishimoto T (2000) c-Mos forces the mitotic cell cycle to undergo meiosis II to produce haploid gametes. PNAS 97:14301–14306

Tong ZB, Gold L, Pfeifer KE, Dorward H, Lee E, Bondy CA, Dean J, Nelson LM (2000) Mater, a maternal effect gene required for early embryonic development in mice. Nat Genet 26:226–227

Tong ZB, Nelson LM (1999) A mouse gene encoding an oocyte antigen associated with autoimmune premature ovarian failure. Endocrinology 140:3720–3726

Yan C, Pendola FL, Jacob R, Lau AL, Eppig JJ, Matzuk MM (2001) *Oospl* encodes a novel mouse oocyte-secreted protein. Genesis 31: 105–110

Yan C, Wang P, DeMayo J, DeMayo F, Elvin J, Carino C, Prasad S, Skinner S, Dunbar B, Dube J, Celeste A, Matzuk M (2001) Synergistic roles of bone morphogenetic protein 15 and growth differentiation factor 9 in ovarian function. Mol Endocrinol 15:854–866

6 The Biochemistry of Oocyte Maturation

S.M. Downs

6.1 Introduction 81
6.2 Maintenance of Meiotic Arrest 82
6.3 Meiotic Induction – A Loss of Inhibition or Positive Stimulation? . 85
6.4 Possible Metabolic Pathways Involved in Hormone-Induced Maturation 88
6.5 AMP-Activated Protein Kinase – A Potential Role in Meiotic Induction 90
6.6 Model for Meiotic Induction 92
6.7 Conclusions 94
References 95

6.1 Introduction

Oocyte maturation is a complex process that encompasses growth and differentiation of the oocyte, acquisition of meiotic competence, initiation and completion of nuclear maturation, and cytoplasmic changes related to fertilizability and post-fertilization developmental potential. The oocyte develops within a syncytial environment, being intimately coupled to the entire somatic compartment of the follicle via granulosa-oocyte and granulosa–granulosa gap junctions (Larsen and Wert 1988). This condition provides an efficient delivery system through which small molecular weight nutritional and regulatory signals can reach the developing oocyte. As the oocyte grows, it continuously stockpiles macromolecules needed for later development, and near the end of its growth phase, the oocyte completes the biochemical changes required to achieve meiotic competence, a condition that supports the resumption of meiosis beyond prophase I. Once oocytes achieve meiotic competence, they are maintained in a prophase I-arrested, germinal vesicle stage until stimulated to resume maturation, either by the preovulatory gonadotropin surge or by follicular atresia. The former stimulus produces developmentally competent ova while the latter condition leads to degenerating oocytes trapped within anovulatory follicles. Meiotic progression beyond the germinal vesicle stage requires the activation of maturation, or M phase, promoting factor (MPF), a heterodimeric protein complex composed of a 34-kDa kinase and 45-kDa cyclin regulatory subunit. Control of the activity of MPF is an essential component of the system regulating both meiotic arrest and meiotic resumption, since this kinase is the driving force behind cell division. Following meiotic resumption (initially manifested by germinal vesicle breakdown), maturation proceeds through extrusion of the first polar body and formation of the second metaphase spindle (MII), where the oocyte arrests for a second time until activated by fertilization. For the purpose of this review, maturation will be defined as the process of meiosis reinitiation; the focus will be on regulation of the immature, germinal vesicle stage, with particular emphasis on how the oocyte is stimulated to resume meiotic maturation.

6.2 Maintenance of Meiotic Arrest

The entire complement of granulosa cells within the follicle appears essential for the proper maintenance of meiotic arrest. Fully grown oocytes within preovulatory follicles that are cultured in hormone-free medium remain in the immature germinal vesicle stage, while cumulus cell-enclosed or denuded oocytes isolated from similar follicles and cultured under identical conditions spontaneously resume nuclear maturation. The cumulus cells are thus incapable of delivering enough endogenous inhibitor to sustain meiotic arrest. Such spontaneous germinal vesicle breakdown is an artifact of experimental manipulation and does not reflect the full complement of biochemical changes occurring during normal maturation conditions, since meiotic resumption in vivo within healthy follicles requires an external hormonal stimulus and active participation of the somatic compartment.

An inhibitory follicular influence originates both from the granulosa cells and from follicular fluid, which accumulates in antral follicles as a composite of blood exudate and follicular secretions. It is not known if the spontaneous maturation that ensues in oocytes after culture in inhibitor-free medium is a result of isolation from the follicular fluid or separation from the bulk of the granulosa cell population or both. Since the meiotically competent oocyte is bathed in follicular fluid, extensive effort has been made to identify potential physiological inhibitors of meiosis within this milieu. Many studies have shown that follicular fluid suppresses the spontaneous maturation of oocytes. To date, the most prominent compounds implicated have been a low molecular weight peptide (Tsafriri 1988) and the purines hypoxanthine and adenosine (Downs et al. 1985; Eppig et al. 1985). Other potential inhibitors include steroids and fatty acids. These inhibitory compounds are likely produced locally and either modify, or interact with, cyclic adenosine monophosphate (cAMP) to achieve meiotic arrest. This idea is supported by the fact that follicular fluid synergizes dramatically with cAMP-elevating agents to block spontaneous germinal vesicle breakdown (Chari et al. 1983; Downs and Eppig 1984).

The gap junctional coupling pathway is thought to be an important conduit through which inhibitory signals are delivered to the oocyte. For example, hypoxanthine is only very poorly taken up by the denuded oocyte but readily accumulates in the cumulus cell-enclosed oocyte (Downs et al. 1986). Hence, in this way granulosa cells can facilitate an inhibitory action of hypoxanthine (as well as other agents) on meiotic maturation by promoting its acquisition by the oocyte. Indeed, denuded oocytes often exhibit higher frequencies of maturation than do oocytes encompassed by cumulus granulosa cells when cultured in inhibitory medium (cf., Schultz et al. 1983a,b; Racowsky 1985a,b). In addition, treating cumulus cell- or follicle-enclosed oocytes with gap junctional blockers can prevent meiotic arrest (Dekel and Piontkewitz 1991; Downs 1995b, 2001), presumably by interfering with gap junction-mediated delivery of inhibitor(s). In an interesting study in hamsters, Racowsky and Baldwin (1989) showed that physical separation of oocyte–cumulus complexes within intact follicles eliminated the meiotic arrest, and this effect was prevented by reassociation with granulosa cells.

A vast literature indicates that elevated levels of cAMP effectively block meiotic resumption in mammalian oocytes. cAMP analogs or cAMP-elevating agents prevent meiotic resumption, while cAMP antagonists have the opposite effect (cf., Downs 1995a). A decrease in oocyte cAMP is associated with germinal vesicle breakdown, and preventing this change interferes with meiotic resumption (Schultz et al. 1983a,b; Vivarelli et al. 1983; Aberdam et al. 1987). Activation of cAMP-dependent protein kinase, or protein kinase A (PKA), mediates the action of cAMP, leading to phosphorylations that bring about meiotic arrest (Schultz 1986). Of interest was the finding that different isoforms of PKA reside in the oocyte and cumulus cells and provide differential control of the oocyte's meiotic status: activation of type I in the oocyte is inhibitory, while activation of type II in the cumulus oophorus leads to meiotic resumption (Downs and Hunzicker-Dunn 1995). cAMP can therefore have paradoxical effects on oocyte maturation, with meiotic status determined by the level of cAMP reached and the duration of the cAMP flux (Dekel et al. 1988).

The effects of protein kinase C (PKC) on oocyte maturation have also been extensively investigated and have been found to closely parallel those of PKA. Activation of the kinase in oocytes suppresses spontaneous nuclear maturation in a wide variety of species; however, activation within follicles or oocyte–cumulus complexes stimulates germinal vesicle breakdown (reviewed by Downs et al. 2001a). Again, the site of stimulation appears to determine the meiotic outcome, with PKC activity in the somatic compartment capable of generating a positive effect that overrides a direct inhibitory effect of the kinase within the oocyte. Gaining an understanding of the potential involvement of PKC in meiotic regulation is somewhat more daunting than that of PKA, however, in the sense that over 11 PKC isoforms have been identified. Nevertheless, the generality of the inhibitory PKC effect suggests an important basic function in meiotic regulation and raises the possibility that PKA and PKC act cooperatively to maintain meiotic arrest.

6.3 Meiotic Induction – A Loss of Inhibition or Positive Stimulation?

The mechanism of meiotic induction in mammalian oocytes has been a difficult puzzle to decipher, and this stems from the fact that both the germ and somatic follicular compartments participate, each with unique physiological and metabolic characteristics. Since these two compartments are so intimately associated and interact so closely with one another, it is often a challenge to pinpoint the critical site of activity of a particular molecule implicated in the induction process.

There are two major mechanisms that have been proposed for the induction of meiotic resumption in mammals: (1) loss of inhibition and (2) generation of a positive stimulus. Of central importance in the first proposed mechanism is that the follicular syncytium provides a means to efficiently deliver small molecular weight inhibitory substances from the somatic compartment to the oocyte. It also incorporates the fact that a progressive mucification and disaggregation of the granulosa cells occurs following the preovulatory gonadotropin surge that uncouples the oocyte from the granulosa cell population. It has been proposed that gap junctional uncoupling during this period, either between granulosa cells or between granulosa cells and the oocyte, interrupts a unidirectional flow of inhibitory cAMP from granulosa cells to the oocyte. Such compromised cAMP transfer results in lower oocyte cAMP levels, reduced PKA activity and, consequently, germinal vesicle breakdown (Dekel and Beers 1978, 1980).

For this first mechanism to be credible, the loss of inhibitory input should occur well before the resumption of nuclear maturation. Structural changes in gap junctions have been reported at the time of, or just prior to, germinal vesicle breakdown (Larsen et al. 1986, 1987; Racowsky et al. 1989; Wert and Larsen 1990), although gap junctional morphology may not always be an accurate indicator of patency (Phillips and Dekel 1991). Measurement of metabolic coupling using radioactive compounds has produced conflicting data regarding the kinetics of uncoupling, as it relates to meiotic resumption. Many studies, in fact, show no significant decline in the coupling index between oocytes and cumulus cells prior to germinal vesicle breakdown in a variety of species. It is possible, however, that of prime importance is the coupling status between the cumulus oophorus and the membrana granulosa, and that uncoupling at this site, despite persistent coupling between oocyte and cumulus cells, would still deny the oocyte inhibitory input, as suggested by Larsen et al. (1987). Nevertheless, if one assumes that cAMP is the inhibitory substance transferred between follicular compartments, a previous study provided evidence inconsistent with this idea. When equine chorionic gonadotropin-primed mice were treated with an ovulatory dose of human chorionic gonadotropin (hCG), cAMP levels in the oocyte–cumulus cell complex continued to rise while germinal vesicle breakdown was occurring, even though oocyte-cumulus cell coupling was maintained at constant levels during this period (Eppig and Downs 1988). Thus, the increased cAMP generated in the cumulus cells was presumably readily accessible to the oocyte through the gap junctional pathway and yet the oocyte still resumed maturation.

The second proposed mechanism, and one that our laboratory has embraced more enthusiastically, involves production by the granulosa compartment of a positive, meiosis-inducing substance in response to gonadotropin stimulation that triggers germinal vesicle breakdown in the continuing presence of meiotic inhibitor. Initial experiments in support of this mechanism showed that cumulus cell-enclosed, but not denuded, oocytes maintained in meiotic arrest with cAMP analogs or inhibitors of cAMP phosphodiesterase could be induced to resume maturation in response to gonadotropin (Dekel and Beers 1978; Downs et al. 1988). A wide variety of ligands has been shown to stimulate maturation in isolated oocyte–cumulus cell complexes in such a manner and include follicle-stimulating hormone, epidermal growth factor, mitogenic lectins, phorbol ester, and cholera toxin (reviewed in Downs 1995a). The lack of effect of these ligands on denuded oocytes indicates that the somatic compartment plays a critical role in mediating meiotic induction; it also suggests that ligand stimulation does not trigger germinal vesicle breakdown simply by removing inhibitory input from the somatic cells.

Whereas the first mechanism considers gap junctions crucial in delivering inhibitory signals, the second mechanism also incorporates the coupling pathway as an essential component, but, instead, as the means for transmitting a stimulatory signal to the oocyte. Hence, it is proposed that an inducing signal, generated in the cumulus/granulosa cells in response to ligand stimulation, traverses the gap junctions to reach the oocyte and bring about meiotic resumption. In support of this, gap junction blockers such as alkanols and β-glycyrrhetinic acid have been shown to prevent the gonadotropin-induced maturation of isolated cumulus cell-enclosed oocytes (Fagbohun and Downs 1991; Coskin and Lin 1994; Downs 1995b, 2001).

An alternative mode of action is for a positive meiosis-inducing substance, produced by the somatic compartment, to be secreted into the extracellular space to act on the oocyte in paracrine fashion. One such compound is meiosis-activating sterol, or MAS. In 1995, Byskov et al. reported the isolation of MAS from bull testis and follicular fluid and proposed that these compounds were natural meiosis inducers in vivo due to their ability to stimulate germinal vesicle breakdown in hypoxanthine-arrested mouse oocytes, and this finding was confirmed in many subsequent studies (e.g., Ruan et al. 1998; Grondahl et al. 1998, 2000; Cavilla et al. 2001). In support of this paracrine effect, cocultured cumulus cells have been found to trigger oocyte maturation in denuded oocytes, presumably by the release of such a diffusible factor (Downs and Mastropolo 1994; Guoliang et al. 1994; Byskov et al. 1997; Downs 2001).

Although much evidence has accumulated to support MAS as a natural meiosis inducer, considerable data also exist that are inconsistent with such a role. For example:

1. MAS is not as effective in cumulus cell-enclosed oocytes as it is in denuded oocytes (Grondahl et al. 1998; Downs et al. 2001b). Since oocytes remain coupled to their cumulus cells up until the time of meiotic resumption, this suggests that oocytes in their native state are less responsive to the sterol.
2. The kinetics of denuded oocyte maturation under optimal MAS-stimulating conditions are attenuated by at least several hours when compared to the kinetics in vivo in response to an ovulatory hCG dose (Hegele-Hartung et al. 1999; Downs et al. 2001b).
3. Inhibitors of sterol synthesis block progesterone production in luteinizing hormone (LH)-treated rat follicles but do not prevent hormone-induced germinal vesicle breakdown (Tsafriri et al. 1998).
4. The timing of lanosterol 14α-demethylase expression during hormone-induced oocyte maturation and its localization within rat follicles were incompatible with a role in meiotic induction (Vaknin et al. 2001).

5. The timing of MAS accumulation in the ovaries of superovulated mice appears not to be tied to meiotic resumption but, rather, to ovulation (Baltsen 2001).

Thus, while MAS is an intriguing molecule that may provide important answers regarding the regulation of meiosis, its function as a physiological meiotic trigger remains inconclusive.

6.4 Possible Metabolic Pathways Involved in Hormone-Induced Maturation

The isolated rodent oocyte–cumulus cell complex has become a popular model system to evaluate the regulation of meiotic induction. Oocytes maintained in the germinal vesicle stage by an inhibitor, often hypoxanthine, are then treated with follicle-stimulating hormone (FSH) to trigger meiotic resumption. FSH is chosen over LH/hCG as the meiotic activator due to a dearth of receptors for these latter hormones on cumulus cells (Eppig et al. 1997). The culture medium can then be modified, or the stimulated oocytes can be treated with one of a variety of pharmacological compounds, to determine what biochemical pathways are involved in this process. The following are a representative sampling of pathways that have been implicated in meiotic resumption using this model system.

6.4.1 Pentose Phosphate Pathway

We discovered about 10 years ago that removing glucose from the culture medium dramatically reduced the meiotic resumption stimulated by FSH (Fagbohun and Downs 1992), and this was confirmed in subsequent studies (Downs and Mastropolo 1994; Downs et al. 1996). Further work showed that FSH-induced maturation was associated with increased hexokinase activity (Downs et al. 1996) and was dependent on glucose metabolism through the pentose phosphate pathway (Downs et al. 1998; Downs and Utecht 1999). This latter finding was important because the end product of the pentose phosphate pathway is phosphoribosylpyrophosphate, the starting substrate for de novo purine synthesis (see below).

6.4.2 De Novo Purine Synthetic Pathway

Although purines have been implicated as physiologically important inhibitors of meiotic maturation, these compounds also have an important function in meiotic induction. De novo purine synthesis is increased by 150% in FSH-treated oocyte–cumulus cell complexes, and such stimulation is prevented by inhibitors of de novo purine synthesis at concentrations that significantly suppress FSH-induced germinal vesicle breakdown (Downs 1997). The means by which increased purine nucleotide synthesis leads to meiotic induction has not been elucidated, but it is probably related to increased, sustained levels of cAMP. The discovery of the involvement of purine synthesis in meiotic induction provided evidence for an extended induction pathway linking the metabolism of an energy substrate, glucose, with the generation of nucleotides (both GTP and ATP) that participate in cAMP dynamics.

6.4.3 Phosphoinositide Pathway

Phosphoinositides are part of an important second messenger system in which stimulation of phospholipase C leads to generation of inositol triphosphate (IP_3), a calcium-releasing ligand, and diacylglycerol, a potent activator of PKC. There is evidence for the participation of both arms of this system in meiotic induction. Microinjection of IP_3 into oocytes has been shown to stimulate or accelerate germinal vesicle breakdown (Homa et al. 1991; Pesty et al. 1994), and calcium ionophores are potent stimulators of oocyte maturation (Tsafriri and Bar-Ami 1978; Powers and Paleos 1982; Racowsky 1986). Coticchio and Fleming (1998) found that either inhibition of phosphoinositide metabolism with neomycin or chelation of intracellular calcium blocked FSH-induced maturation in mouse oocytes. As discussed above, PKC has also been shown to have profound effects on oocyte maturation, and in the mouse these actions are very similar to those of PKA (Downs et al. 2001a).

6.4.4 MAP Kinase Pathway

Mitogen-activated protein (MAP) kinases are activated by a wide variety of external stimuli, commonly operating downstream of growth factors and cytokines. These kinases have a protracted control system, with many different pathways potentially converging to participate in their regulation. In the oocyte, MAPK activity is controlled by p39^{mos} kinase, but MAPK in the somatic compartment has different activating systems. Although many studies have demonstrated that spontaneously maturing oocytes exhibit increased levels of MAPK activity, only limited work has been carried out to assess the possible role of MAPK during meiotic induction. Su et al. (2001) found that treatment of mouse cumulus cell-enclosed oocytes with inhibitors of MAPK activation prevented FSH-induced maturation, thereby implicating MAPK in the induction process. However, the critical site of action could not be determined, since activity increased in both the cumulus cells and oocyte prior to germinal vesicle breakdown. Recent follow-up work by Su et al. (J. Eppig, personal communication) has shown that FSH-induced maturation is not compromised in cumulus cell-enclosed oocytes from *Mos*$^{-/-}$ mice, which contain no active MAPK, indicating that MAPK is not required for this response. Yet, MAPK inhibitors block hormone-mediated MAPK activation and meiotic resumption in cumulus cell-enclosed oocytes from both *Mos*$^{-/-}$ and *Mos*$^{+/+}$ mice, suggesting a requirement for MAPK activity within the cumulus cells in the induction process.

6.5 AMP-Activated Protein Kinase – A Potential Role in Meiotic Induction

There is general support for the idea that a decrease in oocyte cAMP precedes, and is required for, the resumption of nuclear maturation. To accomplish this, cells contain one or more isoforms of cAMP phosphodiesterase (PDE), an enzyme that cleaves the cyclic nucleotide phosphodiester bond to form 5′-AMP. The loss in cAMP lowers PKA activity, which presumably leads to meiotic resumption. Type 3 PDE mRNA expression within rat and mouse oocytes has been reported (Tsafriri et al. 1996; Shitsukawa et al. 2001), and PDE3-specific inhibitors have been shown to block spontaneous oocyte maturation (Tsafriri et al. 1996; Shitsukawa et al. 2001) and, even more importantly, hCG-induced maturation in vivo (Wiersma et al. 1998). Thus, convincing data suggest that the activity of PDE3 within the oocyte is absolutely essential in hormone-induced maturation.

At the time germinal vesicle-stage oocytes are isolated from fully grown antral follicles, it is assumed that cAMP levels are sufficient to maintain meiotic arrest. Hence, in order for meiosis to resume, one would expect a decline in cAMP below this inhibitory threshold and a subsequent lowering of PKA activity. However, there are numerous instances in the literature where, following a particular experimental manipulation, a transient rise, and then decline, in cAMP can occur in the oocyte without levels falling below the freshly isolated value, yet germinal vesicle breakdown ensues. The common factor in these circumstances appears to be a drop in cAMP levels.

While such findings support the importance of PDE in the induction process, they are hard to reconcile with the idea that meiotic resumption is principally due to a significant loss in PKA activity. An important clue may be the seemingly innocuous AMP that results from PDE action. Previously assumed to be a harmless byproduct of cAMP degradation, AMP may actually be an important physiological stimulator of nuclear maturation, due to its ability to activate an important regulatory enzyme, AMP-activated protein kinase (AMPK).

AMPK is a member of the AMPK/SNF1 protein kinase family that is present in a wide variety of organisms. It is a stress response enzyme that normally acts to monitor cellular fuel conditions, being activated by increases in the AMP/ATP ratio, and responds to energy deficits by turning off anabolic lipid and carbohydrate pathways to conserve ATP and turning on the corresponding catabolic pathways to produce more (Hardie and Carling 1997; Winder and Hardie 1999). This is accomplished both by direct phosphorylation of metabolic enzymes and by increases in gene expression (Winder and Hardie 1999; Hardie and Hawley 2001).

A recent study from our lab has examined a potential role for AMPK in meiotic resumption (Downs et al. 2002). Western analysis demonstrated the presence of AMPK catalytic subunits in the mouse oocyte. To determine if AMPK activity could stimulate germinal vesicle breakdown, we utilized the adenosine analog, 5-aminoimidazole-4-carboxamide 1-β-d-ribofuranoside (AICA riboside), which is taken up by cells and phosphorylated by adenosine kinase to the AMP analog, AICA ribotide, a potent activator of AMPK (Sullivan et al. 1994). AICA riboside was an extremely effective stimulator of meiotic resumption and was more active in denuded oocytes than in cumulus cell-enclosed oocytes, suggesting the oocyte as a primary site of action. Coincident with stimulation of meiotic resumption was an increase in the activity of AMPK in extracts of AICA riboside-stimulated oocytes. Moreover, maturation was stimulated by AICA riboside when meiotic arrest was maintained with a wide variety of inhibitors, including hypoxanthine, guanosine, dbcAMP, 8-AHA-cAMP and milrinone. The finding that AICA riboside reversed the inhibitory action of milrinone, a PDE3-specific inhibitor, shows that the need for PDE activity can be bypassed. AICA riboside was, however, ineffective when meiotic arrest was maintained by olomoucine or roscovitine, two inhibitors of MPF. These results suggest that, in mouse oocytes, AMPK acts downstream of PDE but upstream of MPF.

6.6 Model for Meiotic Induction

Figure 1 shows a proposed scheme for meiotic induction in mice that incorporates the findings of numerous studies. It should be emphasized that this is a hypothetical model, and at the moment is restricted to the mouse, with many aspects yet to be confirmed by experimentation.

In the somatic compartment, hormone binding stimulates the production of cAMP via membrane-associated adenylate cyclase. This process is aided by glucose, which is metabolized to adenyl and guanyl nucleotides and perhaps other metabolites (?) that also contribute to cAMP accumulation. The cAMP probably also feeds back in a positive manner to promote these glucose-metabolizing pathways. A protracted cAMP response may be essential for optimal meiotic induction.

cAMP serves as the penultimate second messenger that turns on other pathways such as those that phosphorylate, and thereby activate, MAPK or other kinases. Such activation leads to the generation of a positive stimulus that diffuses down a concentration gradient and enters the oocyte through the gap junctional pathway. The increase in cAMP may also activate the sterol biosynthetic pathway and lead to MAS

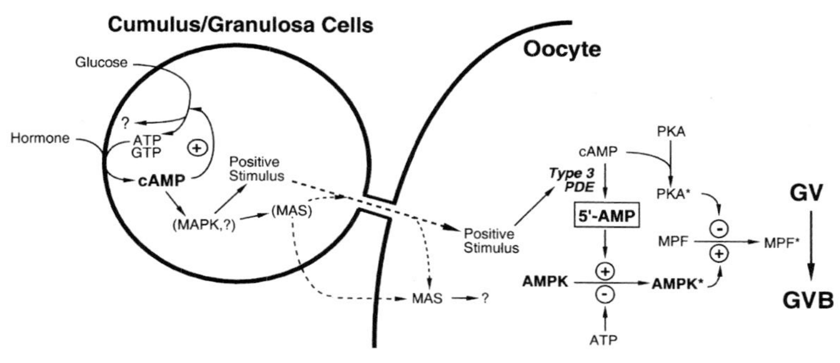

Fig. 1. Proposed model for meiotic induction in mice. Hormone binding to the granulosa cells produces, through a cAMP-dependent pathway, a positive stimulus that traverses gap junctions to activate PDE3 within the oocyte. This results in the degradation of cAMP, which inactivates PKA but simultaneously activates AMPK via generation of AMP. The combined loss of PKA activity but gain in AMPK activity leads to stimulation of MPF and germinal vesicle breakdown (*GVB*). Note that since AMPK is activated by an increase in the AMP/ATP ratio, such activation can be antagonized by increases in ATP. In this model, MAS can be produced in the somatic compartment in response to gonadotropin stimulation, and may enter the oocyte either through gap junctions or by paracrine means, but it is not the principal stimulus driving meiotic resumption. The *asterisk* denotes the active state of the respective kinase

accumulation. We propose that MAS is separate from the positive stimulus and has the potential to reach the oocyte through the gap junctional pathway or by a paracrine route.

The identity of the positive stimulus is unknown, but once threshold levels of the stimulus are reached within the oocyte, type 3 PDE is stimulated. As a result, cAMP levels decline and PKA activity is suppressed. At the same time, AMP is produced, which activates AMPK and provides a direct, positive stimulus for meiotic resumption. Germinal vesicle breakdown (GVB) can therefore occur from the combined loss of the PKA inhibitory influence and increased activity of the meiotic trigger, AMPK. Each of these events independently leads to activation of MPF, which is required for nuclear maturation. However, it should be noted that GVB may be induced by AMPK even with a high background level of PKA activity. This is consistent with the ability of gonadotropins to stimulate meiotic induction in isolated cumulus cell-enclosed oocytes maintained in meiotic arrest with high concentrations of cAMP analogs. It also would explain why a transient rise and fall in oocyte cAMP may induce meiotic resumption even though the cAMP fails to fall below the fresh, presumably inhibitory, level; under these circumstances, the critical event is not a block in PKA activity, but, rather, an increase in the AMP/ATP ratio to an extent sufficient to stimulate AMPK. This could be accomplished by generation of AMP through cAMP PDE activity, consumption of ATP, or a combination of these two processes.

6.7 Conclusions

Meiotic regulation in mammals remains an important unresolved issue in reproductive biology. The need for a syncytial follicular unit, comprising heterologous cell types with disparate metabolic and biochemical potential, constitutes a unique challenge for researchers. Compounding the problem are the differential effects a particular agent may have on meiotic maturation, depending whether it acts in the oocyte or in the granulosa cell. Since spontaneous and hormone-induced maturation occur by different biochemical mechanisms, the use of an in vitro induction paradigm, employing isolated cumulus cell-enclosed oocytes, cultured follicles, or both, will be essential in elucidating the mechanism(s) involved. The basic model of meiotic induction proposed herein incorporates a positive stimulus generated in the somatic compartment in response to gonadotropin binding that traverses the gap junctional communication pathway to stimulate PDE3 activity within the oocyte. The resultant drop in oocyte cAMP leads to meiotic resumption through a two-tiered process involving loss of PKA activity and an increase in AMPK activity. Although many aspects of this model have yet to be demonstrated, it is hoped that such a model provides an impetus for further experimentation that will lead to a better understanding of meiotic regulation.

References

Aberdam E, Hanski E, Dekel N (1987) Maintenance of meiotic arrest in isolated rat oocytes by the invasive adenylate cyclase of Bordetella pertussis. Biol Reprod 36:530–535

Baltsen M (2001) Gonadotropin-induced accumulation of 4,4-dimethylsterols in mouse ovaries and its temporal relation to meiosis. Biol Reprod 65:1743–1750

Byskov AG, Andersen CY, Nordholm L, Thogersen H, Xia G, Wassman O, Andersen JV, Guddal E, Roed T (1995) Chemical structure of sterols that activate oocyte meiosis. Nature 374:559–562

Byskov AG, Andersen CY, Hossaini A, Guoliang X (1997) Cumulus cells of oocyte-cumulus complexes secrete a meiosis-activating substance when stimulated with FSH. Mol Reprod Dev 46:296–305

Cavilla JL, Kennedy CR, Baltsen M, Klentzeris LD, Byskov AG, Hartshorne GM (2001) Effects of meiosis activating sterol (MAS) upon in vitro maturation and fertilization of human oocytes from stimulated and unstimulated ovaries. Hum Reprod 16:547–555

Chari S, Hillensjo T, Magnusson C, Sturm G, Daume E (1983) In vitro inhibition of rat oocyte meiosis by human follicular fluid fractions. Arch Gynecol 233:155–164

Coskun S, Lin YC (1994) Effects of transforming growth factors and activin-A on in vitro porcine oocyte maturation. Mol Reprod Dev 38:153–159

Coticchio G, Fleming S (1998) Inhibition of phosphoinositide metabolism or chelation of intracellular calcium blocks FSH-induced but not spontaneous meiotic resumption in mouse oocytes. Dev Biol 203:201–209

Dekel N, Beers WH (1978) Rat oocyte maturation in vitro: relief of cyclic AMP inhibition by gonadotropins. Proc Natl Acad Sci USA 75:4369–4373

Dekel N, Beers WH (1980) Development of the rat oocyte : inhibition and induction of maturation in the presence or absence of the cumulus oophorus. Dev Biol 75:274–254

Dekel N, Piontkewitz Y (1991) Induction of maturation in vitro of rat oocytes by interruption of communication in the cumulus-oocyte complex. Bull Assoc Anat 75:51–54

Dekel N, Galiani D, Sherizly I (1988) Dissociation between the inhibitory and the stimulatory action of cAMP on maturation of rat oocytes (1988) Mol Cell Endocrinol 56:115–121

Downs SM (1995a) Ovulation 2: control of the resumption of meiotic maturation in mammalian oocytes. In: Grudzinskas JG, Yovich JL (eds) Gametes – the oocyte. Cambridge University Press, Cambridge, pp 150–192

Downs SM (1995b) The influence of glucose, cumulus cells, and metabolic coupling on ATP levels and meiotic control in the isolated mouse oocyte. Dev Biol 167:502–512,

Downs SM (1997) Involvement of purine nucleotide synthetic pathways in gonadotropin-induced meiotic maturation in mouse cumulus cell-enclosed oocytes. Mol Reprod Dev 46:155–167

Downs SM (2001) A gap-junction-mediated signal, rather than an external paracrine factor, predominates during meiotic induction in isolated mouse oocytes. Zygote 9:71–82

Downs SM, Eppig JJ (1984) Cyclic adenosine monophosphate and ovarian follicular fluid act synergistically to inhibit mouse oocyte maturation. Endocrinology 114:418–427

Downs SM, Hunzicker-Dunn M (1995) Differential regulation of oocyte maturation and cumulus expansion in the mouse oocyte-cumulus cell complex by site-selective analogs of cyclic adenosine monophosphate. Dev Biol 172:72–85

Downs SM, Mastropolo AM (1994) The participation of energy substrates in the control of meiotic maturation in murine oocytes. Dev Biol 162:154–168

Downs SM, Utecht AM (1999) Metabolism of radiolabeled glucose by mouse oocytes and oocyte-cumulus cell complexes. Biol Reprod 60:1446–1452

Downs SM, Coleman DL, Eppig JJ (1985) Hypoxanthine is the principal inhibitor of murine oocyte maturation in a low molecular weight fraction of porcine follicular fluid. Proc Natl Acad Sci USA 82:454–458

Downs SM, Coleman DL, Eppig JJ (1986) Maintenance of murine oocyte meiotic arrest: uptake and metabolism of hypoxanthine and adenosine by cumulus cell-enclosed and denuded oocytes. Dev Biol 117:174–183

Downs SM, Daniel SAJ, Eppig JJ (1988) Induction of maturation in cumulus cell-enclosed mouse oocytes by follicle-stimulating hormone and epidermal growth factor: evidence for a positive stimulus of somatic cell origin. J Exp Zool 245:86–96

Downs SM, Humpherson PG, Martin KL, Leese HJ (1996) Glucose utilization during gonadotropin-induced meiotic maturation in cumulus cell-enclosed mouse oocytes. Mol Reprod Dev 44:121–131

Downs SM, Humpherson PG, Leese HJ (1998) Meiotic induction in cumulus cell-enclosed mouse oocytes: involvement of the pentose phosphate pathway. Biol Reprod 58:1084–1094

Downs SM, Cottom J, Hunzicker-Dunn M (2001a) Protein kinase C and meiotic regulation in isolated mouse oocytes. Mol Reprod Dev 58:101–115.

Downs SM, Ruan B, Schroepfer GJ Jr (2001b) Meiosis-activating sterol and the maturation of isolated mouse oocytes. Biol Reprod 64:80–89

Downs SM, Hudson ER, Hardie DG (2002) A potential role for AMP-activated protein kinase in meiotic induction in mouse oocytes. Dev Biol 245:200–212

Eppig JJ, Downs SM (1988) Gonadotropin-induced murine oocyte maturation in vivo is not associated with decreased cyclic adenosine monophosphate in the oocyte-cumulus cell complex. Gamete Res 20:125–131

Eppig JJ, Ward-Bailey PF, Coleman DL (1985) Hypoxanthine and adenosine in murine ovarian follicular fluid: concentrations and activity in maintaining oocyte meiotic arrest. Biol Reprod 33:1041–1049

Eppig JJ, Wigglesworth K, Pendola F, Hirao Y (1997) Murine oocytes suppress expression of luteinizing hormone receptor messenger ribonucleic acid by granulosa cells. Biol Reprod 56:976–984

Fagbohun CF, Downs SM (1991) Metabolic coupling and ligand-stimulated meiotic maturation in the mouse oocyte-cumulus cell complex. Biol Reprod 45:851–859

Fagbohun CF, Downs SM (1992) Requirement for glucose in ligand-stimulated meiotic maturation of cumulus cell-enclosed mouse oocytes. J Reprod Fertil 96:681–697

Grondahl C, Ottesen JL, Lessl M, Faarup P, Murray A, Gronvald FC, Hegele-Hartung C, Ahnfelt-Ronne I (1998) Meiosis-activating sterol promotes resumption of meiosis in mouse oocytes cultured in vitro in contrast to related oxysterols. Biol Reprod 58:1297–1302

Grondahl C, Lessl M, Faerge I, Hegele-Hartung C, Wassermann K, Ottesen JL (2000) Meiosis-activating sterol-mediated resumption of meiosis in mouse oocytes in vitro is influenced by protein synthesis inhibition and cholera toxin. Biol Reprod 62:775–780

Guoliang X, Byskov AG, Andersen CY (1994) Cumulus cells secrete a meiosis-inducing substance by stimulation with forskolin and dibutyric cyclic adenosine monophosphate. Mol Reprod Dev 39:17–24

Hardie DG, Carling D (1997) The AMP-activated protein kinase. Fuel gauge of the mammalian cell? Eur J Biochem 246:259–273

Hardie DG, Hawley SM (2001) AMP-activated protein kinase: the energy charge hypothesis revisited. Bioessays (in press)

Hegele-Hartung C, Kuhnke J, Lesl M, Grondahl C, Ottesen J, Beier HM, Eisner S, Eichenlaub-Ritter U (1999) Nuclear and cytoplasmic maturation of mouse oocytes after treatment with synthetic meiosis-activating sterol. Biol Reprod 61:1362–1372

Homa ST, Webster SD, Russell RK (1991) Phospholipid turnover and ultrastructural correlates during spontaneous germinal vesicle breakdown of the bovine oocyte: effects of a cyclic AMP phosphodiesterase inhibitor. Dev Biol 146:461–472

Larsen WJ, Wert S (1988) Roles of cell junctions in gametogenesis and in early embryonic development. Tissue Cell 20:809–848
Larsen WJ, Wert S, Brunner GD (1986) A dramatic loss of cumulus cell gap junctions is correlated with germinal vesicle breakdown in rat oocytes. Dev Biol 113:517–521
Larsen WJ, Wert S, Brunner GD (1987) Differential modulation of rat follicle cell gap junction populations at ovulation. Dev Biol 122:61–71
Pesty A, Lefevre B, Kubiak J, Geraud G, Tesarik J, Maro B (1994) Mouse oocyte maturation is affected by lithium via the polyphosphoinositide metabolism and the microtubule network. Mol Reprod Dev 38:187–199
Phillips DM, Dekel N (1991) Maturation of the rat cumulus-oocyte complex: structure and function. Mol Reprod Dev 28:297–306
Powers RD, Paleos GA (1982) Combined effects of calcium and dibutyryl cyclic AMP on germinal vesicle breakdown in the mouse oocyte. J Reprod Fertil 66:1–8
Racowsky C (1985a) Effect of forskolin on the spontaneous maturation and cyclic AMP content of hamster oocyte-cumulus complexes. J Exp Zool 234:87–96
Racowsky C (1985b) Effect of forskolin on maintenance of meiotic arrest and stimulation of cumulus expansion, progesterone and cyclic AMP production by pig oocyte-cumulus complexes. J Reprod Fertil 74:9–21
Racowsky C (1986) The releasing action of calcium upon cyclic AMP-dependent meiotic arrest in hamster oocytes. J Exp Zool 239:263–275
Racowsky C, Baldwin KV (1989) In vitro and in vivo studies reveal that hamster oocyte meiotic arrest is maintained only transiently by follicular fluid, but persistently by membrana/cumulus cell contact. Dev Biol 134:297–306
Racoswky C, Baldwin KV, Larabell CA, DeMarais AA, Kazilek CJ (1989) Down-regulation of membrana granulosa cell gap junctions is correlated with irreversible commitment to resume meiosis in golden Syrian hamster oocytes. Eur J Cell Biol 49:244–251
Ruan B, Watanabe S, Eppig JJ, Kwoh C, Dzidic N, Pang J, Wilson WK, Schroepfer GJ Jr (1998) Sterols affecting meiosis: novel chemical syntheses and biological activities and spectral properties of the synthetic sterols. J Lipid Res 39:2005–2020
Schultz RM, Montgomery RR, Belanoff JR (1983a) Regulation of mouse oocyte maturation: implication of a decrease in oocyte cAMP and protein dephosphorylation in commitment to resume meiosis. Dev Biol 97:264–273
Schultz RM, Montgomery RR, Ward-Bailey PF, Eppig JJ (1983b) Regulation of oocyte maturation in the mouse: possible roles of intercellular communication, cAMP, and testosterone. Dev Biol 95:294–304
Schultz RM (1986) Molecular aspects of mammalian oocyte growth and maturation. In: Rossant J, Pederson RA (eds) Experimental approaches to mam-

malian embryonic development. Cambridge University Press, Cambridge, pp 195–237

Shitsukawa K, Andersen CB, Richard FJ, Horner AK, Wiersma A, van Duin M, Conti M (2001) Cloning and characterization of the cyclic guanosine monophosphate-inhibited phosphodiesterase PDE3A expressed in mouse oocyte. Biol Reprod 65:188–196

Sullivan JE, Brocklehurst KJ, Marley AE, Carey F, Carling D, Beri RK (1994) Inhibition of lipolysis and lipogenesis in isolated rat adipocytes with AICAR, a cell-permeable activator of AMP-activated protein kinase. FEBS Lett 353:33–36

Tsafriri A (1988) Local nonsteroidal regulators of ovarian function. In: Knobil E, Neill J et al (eds) The physiology of reproduction. Raven Press, New York, pp 527–565

Tsafriri A, Bar-Ami S (1978) Role of divalent cations in the resumption of meiosis of rat oocytes. J Exp Zool 205:293–300

Tsafriri A, Chun SY, Hsueh AJW, Conti M (1996) Oocyte maturation involves compartmentalization and opposing changes of cAMP levels in follicular somatic and germ cells: studies using selective phosphodiesterase inhibitors. Dev Biol 178:393–402

Tsafriri A, Popliker M, Nahum R, Beyth Y (1998) Effects of ketoconazole on ovulatory changes in the rat: implications on the role of a meiosis-activating sterol. Mol Hum Reprod 4:483–489

Vaknin KM, Lazar S, Popliker M, Tsafriri A (2001) Role of meiosis-activating sterols in rat oocyte maturation: effects of specific inhibitors and changes in the expression of lanosterol 14α-demethylase during the preovulatory period. Biol Reprod 64:299–309

Vivarelli E, Conti M, De Felici M, Siracusa G (1983) Meiotic resumption and intracellular cAMP levels in mouse oocytes treated with compounds which act on cAMP metabolism. Cell Differ 12:271–276

Wert S, Larsen WJ (1990) Preendocytotic alterations in cumulus cell gap junctions precede meiotic resumption in the rat cumulus-oocyte complex. Tissue Cell 22:827–851

Wiersma A, Hirsch B, Tsafriri A, Hanssen RGJM, Van de Kant M, Kloosterboer HJ, Conti M, Hsueh AJW (1998) Phosphodiesterase 3 inhibitors suppress oocyte maturation and consequent pregnancy without affecting ovulation and cyclicity in rodents. J Clin Invest 102:532–537

Winder WW, Hardie DG (1999) AMP-activated protein kinase, a metabolic master switch: possible roles in type 2 diabetes. Am J Physiol Metab 40:E1–E10

7 The Structural Basis of Oocyte-Granulosa Cell Communication

D.F. Albertini

7.1 Background 101
7.2 Structural Properties of Transzonal Projections (TZPs) 102
7.3 Developmental Regulation 106
7.4 Outstanding Questions and Conclusions 108
References 109

7.1 Background

The ontogeny of female germ cells in animals encompasses phases of prolonged storage, rapid growth and maturation, and mechanisms for releasing oocytes from the ovary (Wallace and Selman 1990). Ovarian follicles provide the multicellular unit for prolonged storage of oocytes both prior to and during the reproductive lifespan of females. The follicle, formed by the physical interaction of oocytes and granulosa cells, supports the rapid growth and maturation of oocytes (Canipari 1994). To accomplish this, the somatic granulosa cells surrounding the oocyte undergo periodic changes in structure and function that concurrently attend the needs of the developing oocyte and organismal reproductive cyclicity. The physical linkage between female germ cells and the ovarian soma is finally interrupted during the process of ovulation, even though in many animals the oocyte is released with somatic cells attached to the oolemma or investing extracellular matrices (Suzuki et al. 2000). Thus, from both a phylogenetic and ontogenetic perspective, oogenesis clearly involves a protracted period of contact between the oocyte and surrounding follicle cells. The morphological and physiological relevance of oocyte–granulosa cell contact in the mammalian ovary is considered below with reference to the form, composition and functions subserved by specialized structures known as transzonal projections (TZPs).

7.2 Structural Properties of Transzonal Projections (TZPs)

In the mammalian ovary, oocyte–granulosa contacts are evident within primordial follicles and appear to include at least gap junction-types of specializations (Hertig and Adams 1967; Grazul-Bilska et al. 1997). Once folliculogenesis is initiated, the gradual deposition of the zona pellucida at the oocyte cell surface creates a permanent but malleable extracellular matrix barrier between germ cells and ovarian somatic cells for the duration of oogenesis. In order to establish and maintain direct physical contact at this heterocellular interface, specialized properties of granulosa cells have evolved to both breach the zona pellucida and anchor cytoplasmic projections to the oocyte surface. The devices used by granulosa cells to establish a physical conduit for cell communication have been termed TZPs and their origin from somatic granulosa cells has been confirmed morphologically in living and fixed preparations (Fig. 1A). Most of what is known about the structural properties of TZPs derives from earlier electron microscopy studies, but more recently, confocal microscopy has been adopted as a valuable tool to explore three-dimensional aspects of cell organization at the oocyte-granulosa interface.

7.2.1 Ultrastructural Correlates

Initial studies by Anderson and Albertini (1976) defined morphological variations in the organization of TZPs at the oocyte surface in several mammals. For example, in the rhesus monkey ovarian follicle, TZPs were found to terminate upon broad, non-microvillar plasma membrane domains on the oocyte surface. Focal adhesions at these contacts were flanked by small gap junction plaques. Small gap junctions have also

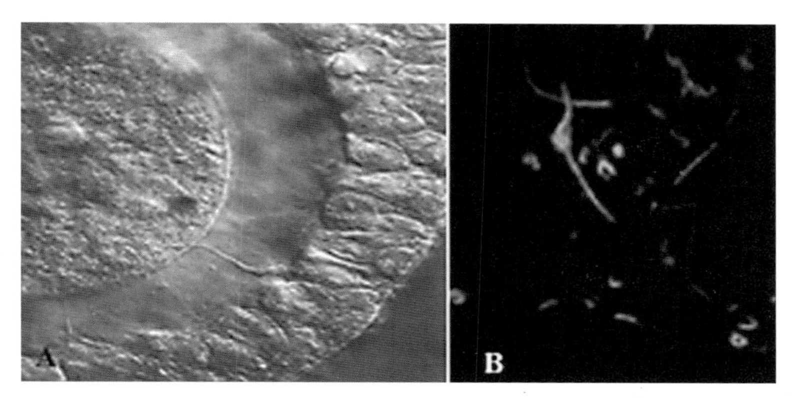

Fig. 1A,B. Transzonal projections (TZP) in living rhesus monkey pre-antral follicle (**A**) and fixed human cumulus-oocyte complex (**B**). Note granulosa cell cytoplasmic projection traversing zona pellucida; these structures, imaged by Nomarski differential interference contrast microscopy, periodically retract and extend in association with mitotic events within the follicular epithelium. In **B**, α-acetylated tubulin antibodies have been used to highlight TZPs within the zona pellucida of a human oocyte. Note both extended TZPs and hoops, with the latter most often seen in association with the oocyte surface

been detected between oocyte microvilli and the tips of small-calibre TZPs enriched in actin filaments (see Sect. 7.2.2). Slender actin-laden TZPs appear to be prominent in rodents whereas larger calibre TZPs with broad terminal contacts and zones of adhesion appear to be more typical of primates and ruminants (Allworth and Albertini 1993; Albertini and Rider 1994) including humans (Combelles et al. 2002). Work by Motta et al. (1994) has furthered detailed the ultrastructure of TZPs in humans with particular reference to changes associated with development of the follicle. They report that TZPs of high density exist in pre-antral follicles where they deeply invaginate the oocyte, sometimes penetrating to close proximity of the germinal vesicle. At later stages of follicle development, TZPs were found to more typically terminate at the oocyte surface and appear to gradually diminish in the number per oocyte with advancing stages of follicle development. Clearly, more work is required to define the spatial organization and composition of these structures during oogenesis, but their prevalence in mammalian ovary and variable organization suggests some degree of plasticity exists during follicle development.

7.2.2 Confocal Microscopy Analysis

The ability to localize specific molecules by immunolabelling procedures, in conjunction with the optical sectioning capabilities of confocal microscopy, has materially extended our understanding of the cytoarchitecture of the oocyte–granulosa interface. Collectively, immunolabelling studies and the use of cytoskeletal inhibitors have defined expression patterns and possible functions for the cytoskeleton within TZPs. Actin filaments are organized in parallel arrays throughout the TZPs in all mammalian species studied (Anderson and Albertini 1976; Albertini and Rider 1994). In all cases examined, aggregates of f-actin are concentrated at TZP terminals consistent with a role in stabilizing cell contacts between oocytes and granulosa (Can et al. 1997). Intermediate filaments of the vimentin variety, typically a marker of cells of mesenchymal origin, have been detected in granulosa cells from humans (Czernobilsky et al. 1985), sheep (Gall et al. 1992) and rodents (Albertini and Kravit 1981), and these appear to be abundant within and at the termini of TZPs of intact cumulus oocyte complexes (Gall et al. 1992). It has also been shown in human and sheep that epithelial keratins are co-expressed with vimentin in granulosa cells (Czernobilsky et al. 1985; Gall et al. 1992). The preferential accumulation of these proteins at TZP termini further suggests that more highly differentiated forms of cell adhesion, namely desmosomes, may maintain oocyte–granulosa attachment as physical stresses due to oocyte growth and follicle expansion are increased during folliculogenesis. Since the cytoskeletal inhibitors acrylamide (for intermediate filaments; Gall et al. 1992) and cytochalasin D (for actin filaments; De Smedt and Szollosi 1991) have both been shown to induce meiotic resumption in sheep cumulus–oocyte complexes (COCs), it has been suggested that these cytoskeletal components provide a structural framework for the maintenance and function of cell communication pathways between oocyte and granulosa.

7.2.3 Microtubule Composition

That TZPs also include microtubules (MTs) as a major cytoskeletal component has more recently become clear (Albertini et al. 2001). Previous studies on bovine COCs illustrated that the oriented elongation of TZPs during hormone-induced oocyte maturation was accompanied by a burst of microtubule assembly within cumulus granulosa cells (Allworth and Albertini 1993). Subsequent studies have further detailed aspects of MT organization and dynamics within TZPs during both follicular development and the periovulatory period. For example, studies on mouse oocytes exposed to the phosphodiesterase inhibitor isobutylmethylxanthine suggest that elevation of granulosa cyclic adenosine monophosphate (cAMP) levels results in a dramatic reduction of MT-bearing TZPs (Albertini et al. 2001). Furthermore, recent evaluation of tubulin isoforms within human oocytes demonstrate a stable subset of MTs bearing α-acetylated tubulin epitopes that form hoop-like arrays at the oocyte surface within TZP termini (Combelles et al. 2002; Fig. 1B). This is confirmed by electron microscopy illustrating prominent microtubule tracks within human cumulus cells in association with organelles (Tesarik and Dvorak 1982). Thus, TZPs of two types appear to exist at the oocyte–granulosa interface. Both actin-rich and tubulin-rich TZPs are distinguishable based upon cytoskeletal content and disposition, although whether these distinct structures subserve selective functions remains to be established (Albertini et al. 2001).

From a compositional point of view, MTs consist of traditional heterodimeric subunit isoforms of both α and β epitopes, and these are routinely detected by immunocytochemical studies of TZPs. What remains to be fully elucidated is whether post-translational modifications of tubulin exist that would implicate changes in polymer stability at specific stages of folliculogenesis. α-Acetylated tubulin is seen in TZPs of both COCs and granulosa from pre-antral mouse follicles. A tendency to orient α-acetylated MTs in pre-antral follicles (Albertini et al. 2001) suggests that TZPs are preferentially polarized and stabilized at critical times of development, possibly to mediate vectorial exchange of signalling molecules or as a reflection of unique cell cycle control points required for lineage selection of mural or cumulus phenotypes (Herman and Albertini 1983). Further characterization of MT phenotypes in TZPs will be necessary to establish how dynamic these structures are.

7.2.4 Additional Components of TZPs

The recent demonstration that molecules involved in neurotransmission are localized at the oocyte–granulosa interface (Grosse et al. 2000) lends further credence to the evolving idea that TZPs serve as axon-like conduits for macromolecular exchange (Allworth and Albertini 1993). To date, discriminating markers for a neuronal phenotype have not been systematically tested, with the exception of the above-cited study. However, markers of synaptic transmission machinery, organelle transport and cell-adhesion-based signalling would all be likely candidates for further exploration of the signalling mechanisms operative at the oocyte-granulosa interface (Fagotto and Gambiner 1996).

7.3 Developmental Regulation

Relatively little is known at present as to how the TZP system is modulated throughout the course of follicular development. It does appear that significant species variations exist in both the composition, structure and expression of TZPs (Albertini and Rider 1994; Can et al. 1997). Moreover, there is mounting evidence to suggest that within a given mammalian species, significant variations exist in the organization of TZPs depending upon the stage of follicle development under study. Two broad categories are worth highlighting with reference to TZP remodelling that occurs (1) during the course of folliculogenesis or (2) during the periovulatory period within the COC.

7.3.1 TZP Remodelling During Folliculogenesis

As noted earlier, the studies of Motta revealed variations in TZP organization and density during human ovarian follicle development (Motta et al. 1994). Both variations in the extent of TZP penetration of the oolemma, which diminished with advancing folliculogenesis and TZP density, followed a similar pattern. In other species this has been less well studied from the point of view of TZPs, but considerable evidence suggests that modulation of gap junctions is subject to tight spatial and temporal controls (Grazul-Bilska et al. 1997).

For example, gap junctions exist even prior to zona deposition in primordial follicles at the oocyte–granulosa interface. Numbers of gap junctions at this interface as well as at the granulosa–granulosa interface are clearly up-regulated by oestrogens and follicle-stimulating hormone (FSH) (Burghardt and Matheson 1982). Moreover, a number of studies have extended this work to show transcriptional up-regulation of the major granulosa cell connexin, cxn 43 (Grazul-Bilska et al. 1997). Whether cxn 43 participates directly or indirectly in oocyte–granulosa communication is not entirely clear. Complicating this prospect is the recent finding that in mice, a unique connexin, the oocyte specific cxn 37, appears to mediate oocyte–granulosa gap junction-mediated communication (Carabatsos et al. 2000). Studies on mice in which cxn 37 was disrupted reveal tandem arrest points for oogenesis and folliculogenesis. For oogenesis, growth and meiotic competence acquisition are incomplete in the absence of functional gap junctions. For folliculogenesis, follicles are arrested at the early antral stage and undergo partial luteinization with advancing age. This phenotype suggests the need for gap junctions in order for both compartments to advance developmentally but clearly defines a degree of development that is independent of gap junctions. Interestingly, MT-TZPs are abundant in these animals, demonstrating that the formation and stabilization of these structures does not require functional coupling via gap junctions (D.F. Albertini and M.J. Carabatsos, unpublished observation).

7.3.2 TZP Remodelling During Ovulation

Substantial evidence exists to support the notion that somatic cell coupling to the oocyte, in terms of both structural integrity and signalling, is modified during the periovulatory period. Two general models exist that include (1) the idea that physical uncoupling both removes meiosis-arresting constraints and allows maturation to proceed and (2) the idea that timely inputs to the oocyte, via the luteinizing hormone (LH) surge, stimulate the resumption of meiosis and perhaps modulate the continuation of events that support maturation and the acquisition of developmental competence. While there is little doubt, especially in rodent models, that physical uncoupling due in part to TZP retraction occurs during oocyte maturation and cumulus expansion, the timing of this process and its underlying mechanism remain incompletely understood (Albertini and Rider 1994). Remodelling of the actin cytoskeleton is likely intrinsic to cumulus cell responsiveness to gonadotrophins or other cumulus factors secreted during ovulation. This was shown directly in hamster COCs treated with FSH under conditions that enhanced meiotic maturation (Plancha and Albertini 1994). Both oocyte cortical actin assembly and withdrawal of actin TZPs were necessary remodelling events for maturation to proceed to completion.

In contrast, there is evidence to suggest that withdrawal of actin-TZPs and de novo growth of MT-TZPs underscores stimulation of COCs in other species such as bovine and primates (Allworth and Albertini 1993; Albertini and Rider 1994; Combelles et al. 2002). While the signalling pathways that mediate these distinct forms of cytoskeletal remodelling await definition, it is likely that extension, anchoring and secretion through hormonally regulated subpopulations of the cumulus underlie critical aspects of oocyte quality determination.

7.4 Outstanding Questions and Conclusions

This brief account of the structural basis of oocyte–granulosa cell communication exposes the rudimentary nature of our understanding of the germ–somatic cell interactions within the mammalian ovary. Like neuronal circuitry within the central nervous system, both the form and substance of communication pathways in the ovary emerge as developmentally complex and "homeostatically" plastic cellular arrays. How heterogeneous are TZPs at different stages of follicle development? What distinctions in molecular composition and follicular architecture underlie the changing demands for gametic or granulosa signalling at critical transitions in oogenesis? Are distinct TZPs mediating oocyte growth and maturation or follicle growth and differentiation? Understanding both the formative and substantive factors that mediate these junctional and paracrine modes of cell communication is imperative if gains are to be made in development of new contraceptive strategies or improvements in assisted reproductive technologies.

References

Albertini DF, Kravit NG (1981) Isolation and biochemical characterization of ten-nanometer filaments from cultured ovarian granulosa cells. J Biol Chem 256:2484–2492

Albertini DF, Rider V (1994) Patterns of intercellular connectivity in the mammalian cumulus-oocyte complex. Microsc Res Tech 27:125–133

Albertini DF, Combelles CM, Benecchi E, Carabatsos MJ (2001) Cellular basis for paracrine regulation of ovarian follicle development. Reproduction 121:647–653

Allworth AE, Albertini DF (1993) Meiotic maturation in cultured bovine oocytes is accompanied by remodeling of the cumulus cell cytoskeleton. Dev Biol 158:101–112

Anderson E, Albertini DF (1976) Gap junctions between the oocyte and companion follicle cells in the mammalian ovary. J Cell Biol 71:680–686

Burghardt RC, Matheson RL (1982) Gap junction amplification in rat ovarian granulosa cells. I. A direct response to follicle-stimulating hormone. Dev Biol 94:206–215

Can A, Holmes RM, Albertini DF (1997) Analysis of the mammalian ovary by confocal microscopy. In: Motta PM (ed) Microscopy of reproduction and development: a dynamic approach. Antonio Delfino Editore, Rome, pp 101–108

Canipari R (1994) Cell-cell interactions and oocyte growth. Zygote 2:343–345

Carabatsos MJ, Sellitto C, Goodenough DA, Albertini DF (2000) Oocyte-granulosa cell heterologous gap junctions are required for the coordination of nuclear and cytoplasmic meiotic competence. Dev Biol 226:167–179

Combelles CM, Cekleniak NA, Racowsky C, Albertini DF (2002) Assessment of nuclear and cytoplasmic maturation in in vitro matured human oocytes. Hum Reprod 17:1006–1016

Czernobilsky B, Moll R, Levy R, Franke WW (1985) Co-expression of cytokeratin and vimentin filaments in mesothelial, granulosa and rete ovarii cells of the human ovary. Eur J Cell Biol 37:175–190

De Smedt V, Szollosi D (1991) Cytochalasin D treatment induces meiotic resumption in follicular sheep oocytes. Mol Reprod Dev 29:163–171

Fagotto F, Gumbiner BM (1996) Cell contact-dependent signaling. Dev Biol 180:445–454

Gall L, De Smedt V, Ruffini, S (1992) Co-expression of cytokeratins and vimentin in sheep cumulus-oocyte complexes. Alteration of intermediate filament distribution by acrylamide. Dev Growth Differ 34:579–587

Grazul-Bilska AT, Reynolds LP, Redmer DA (1997) Gap junctions in the ovaries. Biol Reprod 57:947–957

Grosse J, Bulling A, Brucker C, Berg U, Amsterdam A, Mayerhofer A, Gratzl M (2000) Synaptosome-associated protein of 25 kilodaltons in oocytes and steroid- producing cells of rat and human ovary: molecular analysis and regulation by gonadotropins. Biol Reprod 63:643–650

Herman B, Albertini DF (1983) Microtubule regulation of cell surface receptor topography during granulosa cell differentiation. Differentiation 25:56–63

Hertig AT, Adams EC (1967) Studies on the human oocyte and its follicle. I. Ultrastructural and histochemical observations on the primordial follicle stage. J Cell Biol 34:647–675

Motta PM, Makabe S, Naguro T, Correr S (1994) Oocyte follicle cells association during development of human ovarian follicle. A study by high resolution scanning and transmission electron microscopy. Arch Histol Cytol 57:369–394

Plancha CE, Albertini DF (1994) Hormonal regulation of meiotic maturation in the hamster oocyte involves a cytoskeleton-mediated process. Biol Reprod 51:852–864

Suzuki H, Jeong BS, Yang X (2000) Dynamic changes of cumulus-oocyte cell communication during in vitro maturation of porcine oocytes. Biol Reprod 63:723–729

Tesarik J, Dvorak M (1982) Human cumulus oophorus preovulatory development. J Ultrastruct Res 78:60–72

Wallace RA, Selman K (1990) Ultrastructural aspects of oogenesis and oocyte growth in fish and amphibians. J Electron Microsc Tech 16:175–201

8 Ageing and Aneuploidy in Oocytes

U. Eichenlaub-Ritter

8.1 Introduction . . . 111
8.2 Maternal Age-Related Trisomy . . . 112
8.3 Aneuploidy in Human Oocytes and Embryos . . . 115
8.4 Nondisjunction and Predivision in the Genesis of Aneuploidy . . . 117
8.5 Origin of Aneuploidy: Unique Characteristics of Mammalian Oogenesis . . . 118
8.6 Experimental Studies in the CBA/Ca Mouse to Analyse the Origin of Aneuploidy . . . 123
8.7 Cell–Cell Interactions, and Expression and Aneuploidy in Oocytes . . . 128
8.8 Summary and Future Prospects . . . 129
References . . . 130

8.1 Introduction

Correlations between maternal age and Down syndrome have been known already for over half a century (Penrose 1933; Bond and Chandley 1983). Still, the reasons for the dramatic increase in risks for a trisomic conceptus, spontaneous abortion associated with a chromosomally unbalanced embryo and the significantly reduced developmental potential of oocytes and embryos in aged women are unclear. Demographic analysis shows that there still is a trend for delaying childbearing to advanced maternal ages in many industrialized countries. Accordingly, it has been estimated that 25% of conceptions will involve women of 35 years or older in the Netherlands in 2005–2009 (te Velde and

Pearson 2002). Many couples attending the infertility clinics are of advanced age. Therefore, it is important to investigate the origin of the maternal age-related decline in fertility associated with aneuploidy in oocytes in order to predict individual risks and, possibly, improve treatment. This contribution reviews briefly the current status of research on the incidence and the origin of aneuploidy in aged oocytes in humans and some experimental animals. The observations suggest that prenatal events in oogenesis and recombination patterns influence susceptibility of chromosomes to errors in segregation, but that the depletion of the follicle pool, hormonal homeostasis, the oocyte-specific fragility of cohesion between homologues and permissive cell-cycle regulation at maturation may be important in the reduced quality of aged oocytes, which affects critically the fidelity of chromosome segregation and developmental potential.

8.2 Maternal Age-Related Trisomy

Aberrant development and implantation failure of the embryo and high risks for spontaneous abortions are the major causes of reduced fertility with advanced maternal age (Fig. 1a). Thus, a high percentage of spontaneous abortions are aneuploid. Retrospective analysis of the origin of the extra chromosome in trisomic conceptions has shown that the vast majority of extra chromosomes is derived by the oocyte and comes from a failure in separation of homologous chromosomes at meiosis I (Eichenlaub-Ritter 2000; Hassold and Hunt 2001). For instance, 88% of all clinically recognized trisomy 21 cases are of maternal origin, a much lower percentage (8%) is associated with nondisjunction at spermatogenesis and a small portion (3%) is mitotically derived (Lamb et al. 1996, 1997; Eichenlaub-Ritter 2000; Hassold and Hunt 2001) (Fig. 1b). For trisomy 16 it has been shown that clinically recognized cases were exclusively of maternal origin and derived by a first meiotic error (Hassold et al. 1995) (Fig. 1b). An exception is trisomy 18, most of which appears related to a second meiotic error in oogenesis (33% meiosis I versus 56% maternal meiosis II errors; Bugge et al. 1998; Hassold and Hunt 2001). While close to 50% of all XXY cases are associated with an error in segregation of sex chromosomes at spermatogenesis (MacDonald et al. 1994), none of the trisomy 16 cases (Hassold et al. 1995), and only 2.1% of trisomy 18 (Bugge et al. 1998) and 5.4% of the trisomy 21 cases (Lamb et al. 1997), are compatible with a male meiotic error (e.g. Eichenlaub-Ritter 2000). Collectively, trisomy data suggest that loss of fidelity of chromosome segregation at the first meiotic division in the oocyte (Fig. 1a) is the major cause of chromosomal imbalance in the embryo and in spontaneous abortions, stillbirths or a clinically recognized numerical chromosomal aberration in the child (Fig. 1a,b) (Eichenlaub-Ritter 1998; Hassold and Hunt 2001).

While only 5% of all clinically recognized pregnancies of young women (>25 years) are estimated to be trisomic, the rate increases dramatically to 35% and more in 40-year-old women (Hassold and Hunt 2001). Risk for nondisjunction increases generally (Warburton and Kinney 1996), but chromosomes appear to be differentially susceptible to errors in segregation at oogenesis. For instance, the incidence of trisomy 16 increases linearly over all maternal ages, while trisomy 15 and 21 rise in an exponential fashion when women reach the age of 35 or above (Hassold et al. 2000). This and the relative association between trisomy and reduced, absent and high recombination (see below) imply that several mechanisms may contribute to aneuploidy in oocytes. Monosomies are rarely detected in clinically recognized pregnancies except for the sex chromosomes. This appears mainly due to lethality of the state (e.g. due to gene dosage effects). When chromosomal constitution in oocytes and preimplantation embryos is analysed by conventional spreading and staining of chromosomes, hypoploidy rate (less than the usual chromosome numbers) is usually higher as compared to hyperploidy rate (extra chromosomes; see below). However, this may be partially attributed to the loss of chromosomes during spreading rather than errors in segregation. LeMaire Adkins et al. (2000) described a preferential segregation of the single X chromosome in X0 mice to the oocyte and suggested that this was related to intrinsic properties of the spindles in mammalian oocytes. Generally, it may be assumed that age-related aneuploidy in oocytes is derived by both loss and gain of a chromosome (e.g. Márquez et al. 1998).

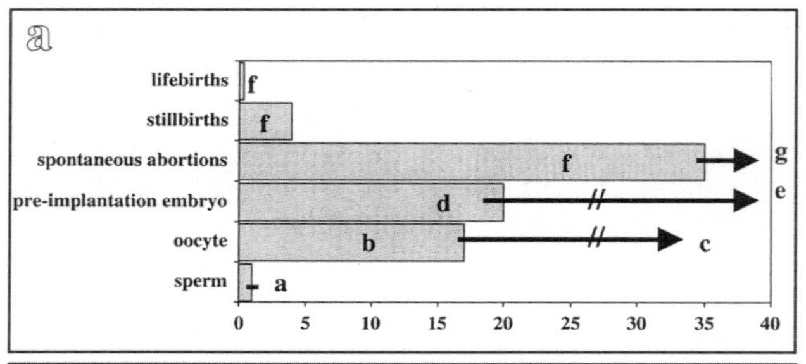
a
lifebirths
stillbirths
spontaneous abortions
pre-implantation embryo
oocyte
sperm
f
f
f
g
d
e
b
c
a
0
5
10
15
20
25
30
35
40

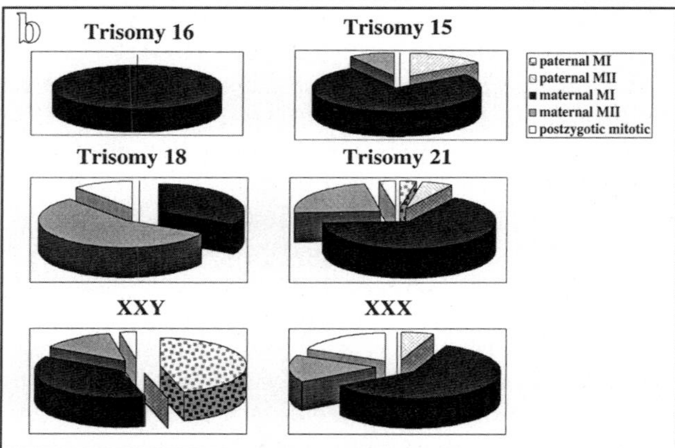
b
Trisomy 16
Trisomy 15
paternal MI
paternal MII
maternal MI
maternal MII
postzygotic mitotic
Trisomy 18
Trisomy 21
XXY
XXX

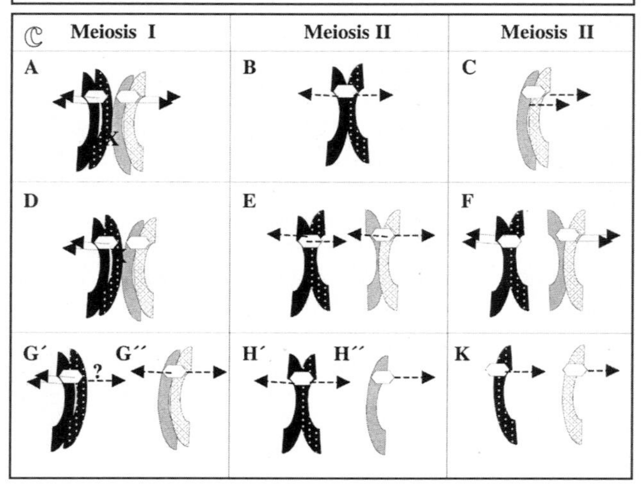
c
Meiosis I
Meiosis II
Meiosis II
A
B
C
D
E
F
G´
G´´
?
H´
H´´
K

8.3 Aneuploidy in Human Oocytes and Embryos

Many oocytes and embryos have become available for cytogenetic analysis in assisted reproduction in recent years. Collecting data on spread human oocytes, which were analysed by conventional staining and banding techniques from the literature between 1985 and 1995, suggests that, on average, 20%–25% of human oocytes are aneuploid (including hypoploids and hyperploids) at metaphase II (Eichenlaub-Ritter 1998). Conservative estimates of aneuploidy, which are based on the assumption that hypoploidy is equally frequent as hyperploidy, suggest that about 17% of all human oocytes from this source may be chromosomally unbalanced (Eichenlaub-Ritter 1996). When taking into account that about 1%–2% of sperm carry a numerical aberration (Hassold and Hunt 2001), and that errors in segregation also occur at anaphase II in the oocyte, on average, about 20% of all human embryos are expected to be aneuploid (Fig. 1a). This agrees well with estimates from trisomy studies (Hassold and Hunt 2001). Rates as high as 20% aneuploidy have also been observed in "spare", normal human embryos from

◄

Fig. 1. a Incidence of aneuploidy in human germ cells and in development. (Data are from: *a*, Hassold 1998; *b*, Eichenlaub-Ritter 1998; *c*, Márquez et al. 1998; Nakaoka et al. 1998; Martini et al. 2000; Verlinski et al. 2001; *d*, Jamieson et al. 1994; *e*, Munné and Cohen 1998; Márquez et al. 2000; *f*, Hassold and Hunt 2001; *g*, Fritz et al. 2001). **b** Origin of extra chromosomes in trisomies. (Data from Hassold and Hunt 2001). **c** Alignment and behaviour of chromosomes and mechanisms that result in errors in chromosome segregation and aneuploidy in oocytes. *A*, Normal reductional segregation of homologues in a bivalent at meiosis I. *B*, Normal equational segregation of sister chromatids at meiosis II. *C*, Classical concept of nondisjunction of sister chromatids at meiosis II. *D*, Classical concept of nondisjunction of homologues at meiosis I. *E*, Equational segregation of sister chromatids following first meiotic nondisjunction. *F*, Aberrant reductional segregation of homologues at meiosis II following a first meiotic nondisjunction event. *G´*, *G´´*, Precocious separation of homologues (or presence of achiasmatic, univalent chromosomes) and random segregation of univalent (*G´*) or premature equational segregation of chromatids at meiosis I instead of meiosis II (*G´´*). *H´*, *H´´*, Segregation of sister chromatids at meiosis II following predivision at meiosis I. *K*, Random segregation of prematurely separated sister chromatids. *Dotted arrows*, reductional segregation; *dashed arrows*, equational segregation. For simplicity, exchanged regions on sister chromatids have been omitted

in vitro fertilization (IVF) and intracytoplasmic sperm injection (ICSI) subjected to spreading and conventional staining/banding techniques (Jamieson et al. 1994). The overall rate of aneuploidy appeared increased in embryos from older patients as compared to younger ones but this was not significant. From over 20 reports on the chromosomal constitution of human oocytes collected between 1985 and 1995, only six found a significant effect of maternal age (Eichenlaub-Ritter 1998). High rates of aneuploidy in oocytes and embryos and the absence of a correlation to maternal age may be related to the source of the material that has been analysed so far. Human oocytes in cytogenetic studies were predominantly unfertilized and acquired from patients of advanced reproductive age obtained from stimulated cycles for various indications. There is so far no evidence that stimulation per se increases aneuploidy significantly in human oocytes (Plachot 2001). Although Gras et al. (1992) found 20% aneuploidy in unstimulated oocytes and 35% and 32% aneuploidy after superovulation with clomiphene citrate/human menopausal gonadotropin (Cl/hMG) or buserelin-flare, the difference was non-significant. Van Blerkom and Davis (2001) observed a progressive and significant increase in defects in spindle structure in metaphase II oocytes from the mouse with repetitive hyperstimulation. Aneuploidy was not analysed. The increase in spindle aberrations only occurred when oocytes matured in vivo and not in vitro, suggesting an influence of the ovarian/follicular environment at maturation on spindle formation. Data from an oocyte donation programme suggest that up to nine stimulation cycles in women of young age do not influence oocyte numbers or quality (Caligara et al. 2001).

Most recent studies employing fluorescent in situ hybridization (FISH) with chromosome-specific probes for up to nine chromosomes found a correlation between maternal age and aneuploidy in oocytes and preimplantation embryos, in agreement with expectations from trisomy data (e.g. Dailey et al. 1996; Benadiva et al. 1996; Benzacken et al. 1998; Gianaroli et al. 1999). Since efficiency of FISH is not 100%, there is a statistical risk to obtain false-positive or -negative results using FISH with single cells. The amazingly high levels of mosaicism (Delhanty et al. 1997; Munné and Cohen 1998; Iwarsson et al. 1999) detected by FISH in blastomeres of spare, aberrant or normal human embryos may partly be related to the reliability of the method. It cannot be excluded that in vitro fertilization and culture affect chromosome segregation. Using comparative genomic hybridization, Wells and Delhanty (2000) showed that mitotic nondisjunction commonly occurs in human preimplantation development in vitro and significantly contributes to aberrant embryos. Lack of cell cycle checkpoints during early embryogenesis could contribute to mosaicism (Harrison et al. 2000). More data are needed from cytogenetic and molecular analysis of human oocytes and polar bodies, as well as from preimplantation genetic diagnosis (PGD), to evaluate the relative contribution of maternal age versus other factors to aneuploidy in oocytes and embryos.

8.4 Nondisjunction and Predivision in the Genesis of Aneuploidy

Angell (1991) detected univalent chromosomes in human oocytes that were donated for research. She postulated that precocious segregation of homologues at meiosis I (predivision) is responsible for aneuploidy in oocytes. Predivision predisposes oocytes to random segregation of the "functional" univalents and/or to a premature separation of chromatids at anaphase I (Fig. 1c). Angell (1997) found a significant correlation between advanced maternal age and single or multiple chromatids in human metaphase II oocytes. Therefore, Wolstenholme and Angell (2000) proposed that precocious separation of centromeres of sister chromatids, in particular in bivalents with a susceptible constitution (e.g. such with only one distal chiasma) are responsible for most maternal age-related trisomies.

It was previously believed that first meiotic errors were based predominantly on random segregation of univalents, or failure of homologues in bivalents to properly orient, or disjoin, such that they did not migrate to opposite spindle poles at anaphase I (Fig. 1c, "D"). According to the "classic" concept, meiosis II errors are induced by nondisjunction of chromatids at anaphase II (Fig. 1c, "C"). Now it appears that predivision of homologues at meiosis I (Fig. 1c, "G´") and precocious segregation of chromatids at first anaphase (Fig. 1c, "G´´") or at metaphase II also contribute to aneuploidy. Single or multiple chromatids, which are not attached to each other at centromeres until anaphase II (Fig. 1c, "K"), have a high risk to randomly segregate (Nasmyth 2001; Lee and Orr-Weaver 2001).

Several studies of human oocytes and polar bodies detected chromatids at metaphase II (e.g. Dailey et al. 1996; Márquez et al. 1998; Nakaoka et al. 1998; Mahmood et al. 2000; Martini et al. 2000; Verlinski et al. 2001; Clyde et al. 2001). However, the percentage of human metaphase II oocytes with chromatids varies widely between individual reports. We have evidence that precocious separation of chromatids may be induced by culture conditions (Betzendahl et al. in preparation). Mailhes et al. (1998) showed in an elegant study in the mouse that the numbers of chromatids at metaphase II became significantly elevated when oocytes aged postovulatory. One-cell zygotes obtained after fertilization of these oocytes had significantly increased rates of aneuploidy. Therefore, ageing at meiosis II predisposes to random chromosome segregation and aneuploidy, in addition to age (Sakurada et al. 1996). Separation of chromatids also occurs frequently and fairly rapidly in the first polar bodies and oocytes of the human during culture after oocyte retrieval. Genetic background appears to influence the relative propensity of univalents in mammalian oocytes to separate their sister chromatids either equationally (sister chromatids segregate to opposite poles/predivision) or reductionally (both sister chromatids segregate to the same pole as in normal bivalents, Fig. 1c, "G´, G''") at first meiosis (LeMaire Adkins et al. 2000; Hodges et al. 2001). Preliminary data from presumably normal, donated human oocytes imply that errors in segregation of whole chromosomes is the predominant cause of aneuploidy in humans, while premature chromatid segregation may occur in only one fifth of cases (Hassold and Hunt 2001).

8.5 Origin of Aneuploidy: Unique Characteristics of Mammalian Oogenesis

8.5.1 Longevity of Oocytes and Selection Processes

Oocytes are among the most long-lived cells in the human body. While the differentiated somatic cells of many tissues have a fairly limited lifespan, and are constantly being replaced by mitotically dividing progenitor cells, oogonia enter S phase already in the embryonal ovary but complete the second meiotic division much later after fertilization in the sexually mature adult woman. The long arrest in dictyate stage of "aged" oocytes has been discussed in the genesis of aneuploidy. If general ageing processes directly affect the quality of the oocyte, for instance, by inducing oxidative damage (e.g. Tarin 1996) and mutations and deletions in DNA of oocytes or mitochondria (e.g. Keefe et al. 1995; Schon et al. 2000), or by affecting mitochondrial function (e.g. Muller-Hocker et al. 1996; Wilding et al. 2001) or cohesion between chromosomes (Wolstenholme and Angell 2000; Hodges et al. 2001), a correlation between chronological age, and aneuploidy in oocytes would be expected. In fact, spindles in human oocytes of aged women often have aberrant spindles and unordered chromosomes (Battaglia et al. 1996; Volarcik et al. 1998). It is feasible that the extremely long arrest of the human oocyte contributes to the exceptionally high susceptibility to aneuploidy in oocytes of our species, while rises in chromosomally unbalanced oocytes in other species like the mouse, the hamster etc. is not that dramatic (Bond and Chandley 1983) due to a relatively shorter time of survival of primordial follicles and oocytes. Still, some observations in humans and experimental animals imply that physiological age may be more important than chronological age.

The pool of oogonia, which become primary oocytes in humans and initiate S phase, comprises about 7 million cells at 4 to 5 months of gestation. Of these, only about 400 oocytes become maximally ovulated over the entire reproductive period (Faddy 2000). Aneuploidy appears to increase exponentially when the primordial follicle pool reaches a critical size. Oocyte and follicle pool size is genetically determined and depends on many factors (for discussion, see Eichenlaub-Ritter and Peschke 2002). For instance, the presence of a pachytene checkpoint (Roeder and Bailis 2000) probably is responsible for apoptosis of many primary oocytes, which are pairing and recombination deficient, thus causing severe depletion of the follicle pool (Woods et al. 1999; Tay and Richter 2001; Vaskivuo et al. 2001; Libby et al. 2002). Critical depletion of the follicle pool close to the end of the reproductive period that influences vascularization (Coulam et al. 1999; Bhal et al. 2001), selection processes (Warburton and Kinney 1996; te Velde and Pearson 2002) and hormonal homeostasis (Crowley et al. 1979; te Velde and Pearson 2002) has been postulated to compromise oocyte quality and fidelity of chromosome segregation. In agreement with this, epidemiological studies showed that women with a trisomy 21 pregnancy tend to reach menopause earlier compared to controls (Kline et al. 2000). Significantly more young women with a trisomy 21 conception had a reduced follicle pool (e.g. by ovarian surgery or absence of an ovary) compared to controls (Freeman et al. 2000). In the CBA/Ca mouse, which has a comparatively small pool of follicles that is depleted by the end of the reproductive period (similar to the human; Fabricant and Schneider 1978), unilateral ovariectomy caused chromosomally aberrant implants at a fairly early maternal age (Gosden 1973; Brook et al. 1984). Disorder in alignment of chromosomes at the metaphase II spindle was increased in spontaneously ovulated oocytes in correlation with depletion of the follicle pool rather than chronological age in unilaterally ovariectomized mice (Eichenlaub-Ritter et al. 1988). Further studies are needed to see whether early age at menopause as a genetic trait or precocious depletion of the follicle pool (e.g. by chemotherapy, lifestyle, or exposure to pollutants) shifts the risk of a woman for aneuploidy in oocytes and for a trisomic conceptus to younger ages.

8.5.2 Constitutive Developmental Arrest in Oogenesis and Permissive Checkpoints

Human spermatogenesis is characterized by low rates of aneuploidy and minor effects of age on meiotic nondisjunction (Hassold 1998). Spermatocytes are continuously progressing through meiosis, while oogenesis is characterized by constitutive meiotic arrest at distinct stages of oocyte development. Meiosis is arrested first in the embryonal ovary, in oocytes that have completed the initial stages of chromosome replication, pairing and recombination. Oocytes acquire meiotic competence during folliculogenesis in the sexually mature woman when follicle and oocyte growth have been completed. After initiation of resumption of maturation, and meiotic progression to metaphase II, oocytes become again constitutively arrested in meiosis at metaphase II until fertilization triggers completion of second meiosis.

Timing during division is controlled by the state of spindle formation and chromosome behaviour in dividing somatic cells and spermatocytes. Only when chromosomes have congressed to the spindle equator, anaphase is initiated. The anaphase promoting factor (APC), a ubiquitin ligase 3 complex, targets proteins for degradation. In mitotic anaphase, degradation of securin frees a separin protease, which cleaves proteins from the cohesion complex holding chromatids together. Disjunction of homologues at meiosis I also depends on cleavage of highly conserved meiotic cohesin proteins (Parisi et al. 1999; Buonomo et al. 2000). APC induces concomitantly the degradation of cyclin B and inactivation of maturation promoting factor (MPF). When chromosomes are not properly aligned or attached to spindle fibres, a checkpoint is triggered, which blocks cells at metaphase (e.g. Nicklas et al. 2001). APC is inactivated by the mitotic checkpoint complex (Gardner and Burke 2000; Sudakin et al. 2001). In this way, the degradation of securin is inhibited. Checkpoint genes are also expressed in meiosis, as recently shown in yeast (Shonn et al. 2000) and human oocytes (Steuerwald et al. 2001). Oocytes will not segregate homologues or chromatids in absence of a spindle (Eichenlaub-Ritter and Boll 1989; Soewarto et al. 1995). However, depolymerization of microtubules by reversible nocodazole treatment during prometaphase I of oogenesis does not cause a delay in the time of anaphase I progression while anaphase I is delayed when oocytes are exposed to a cytostatic drug at metaphase I (Brunet et al. 1999). Therefore, oocytes appear most vulnerable to disturbances for a long period of maturation, and checkpoint control is expressed only after firm attachment of chromosomes to the spindle.

There is a necessity in oogenesis to adjust the meiotic timing to the physiological processes, which are required for fertilization and implantation of the embryo. In the mouse, the length of maturation to anaphase I depends on the expression and turnover of cyclin B (Ledan et al. 2001). Coordination of events, which depend on feedback circuits and which regulate timing of events in oogenesis may therefore be particularly susceptible to reproductive ageing and a relaxed checkpoint control. In a young woman, relaxed checkpoint control is possibly of no consequence because folliculogenesis is well controlled, there are plenty of good follicles for selection and only high quality oocytes are provided to resume maturation. When a normal spindle is formed, chromosome congression can occur in a short period and chromosomes are already aligned when anaphase I is triggered due to a critical reduction in cyclin B. However, when disturbances in spindle formation occur in aged oocytes, which come from developmentally compromised follicles, a relaxed checkpoint control during prometaphase I may allow anaphase progression with unaligned chromosomes (LeMaire-Adkins et al. 1997) and this may pose a great risk for errors in chromosome segregation.

8.5.3 Recombination, Aneuploidy and Maternal Age

Replication of DNA, formation of a synaptonemal complex and pairing and recombination between homologous chromosomes are essential features of early meiosis in the embryonal ovary. Besides an increasing genetic diversity of gametes and recombination between the originally maternally and paternally derived chromosomes, they provide sites of exchange on homologous chromosomes, which maintain physical attachment to chromosomes in bivalents up to anaphase I (Fig. 1c, "A"). The chiasmata hold homologues together and facilitate biorientation of homologues on the first meiotic spindle, which is essential for reductional segregation of chromosomes at anaphase I. Absence of recombination is a risk factor in aneuploidy irrespective of gender and age (e.g. Sears et al. 1992), and the numbers and positioning of chiasmata influence fidelity of chromosome segregation at meiosis (e.g. Koehler et al. 1996). For instance, failure in recombination between the X and Y chromosome significantly contributes to chromosomal imbalance in sperm and sex chromosome aneuploidy in embryos (Hassold et al. 1991). The majority of trisomy 21 at all maternal ages involves achiasmatic chromosomes (Hassold et al. 2000). The relative length of the recombination map, an indicator of frequency of meiotic exchange, is decreased for trisomies 21, which are compatible with a maternal meiosis I error (Hassold and Hunt. 2001). Since the recombination map of the extra chromosome 21 in trisomy 21, which is associated with a meiosis II error, is longer than the normal segregating chromosome, it has been suggested that the majority of nondisjunction events in chromosome segregation of oogenesis, including failure of sister chromatid segregation, are initiated at meiosis I (Lamb et al. 1996).

Henderson and Edwards (1968) reported an age-related increase in univalent chromosomes in aged oocytes of mice and suggested that recombination is reduced in pools of oocytes, which enter meiosis late in the embryonal ovary. Provided these oocytes are also retained in the ovary for the longest period before resuming maturation (according to the existence of a "production line"), univalency would be expected to increase aneuploidy and errors in homologue segregation at anaphase I. For rodents, increases in univalent chromosomes were reported in oocytes (Sugawara and Mikamo 1983), and evidence for a "production line" exists (Polani and Crolla 1981). However, there is no indication that the recombination rate becomes generally reduced with age in humans (Hassold and Hunt. 2001). Furthermore, trisomy 15 appears to involve mostly chromosomes with one exchange in oocytes of younger women. With advanced age of mothers, chromosomes 15 with two and more exchanges also seem susceptible to nondisjunction (Robinson et al. 1998; Hassold et al. 2000). In conclusion, risk for each chromosome to contribute to trisomy with advancing maternal age appears different and preferentially involves certain chromosomal configurations according to the presence and distribution of exchanges. Trisomy data therefore suggest that certain chromosomal configurations (e.g. bivalents with more than two chiasmata) are safely processed in the cytoplasm of a young oocyte but at high risk for aberrant segregation in aged oocytes. This led Lamb et al. (1997) to propose that "two hits" are necessary in the genesis of aneuploidy, the presence of a susceptible chromosome and another disturbance.

8.6 Experimental Studies in the CBA/Ca Mouse to Analyse the Origin of Aneuploidy

8.6.1 Recombination Patterns, Age and Follicle Pool

We used the CBA/Ca mouse as a model to identify susceptible chromosomal conditions and the mechanism behind the second "hit" (G. Michel et al., manuscript submitted). Oocytes were isolated from antral follicles of sexually mature young or aged mice at the same day of the natural cycle (diestrous). They were cultured for 3 h or 6 h in vitro when most oocytes had undergone germinal vesicle breakdown (GVBD) and no bipolar spindle had formed, or when they had reached late prometaphase I and chromosomes were in the process of congression. Since the loss of meiotic proteins, which hold chromosomes together may contribute to errors in chromosome segregation with age (Wolstenholme and Angell 2000; Hodges et al. 2001), we analysed the occurrence of true univalents at 3 h maturation when chromosomes were not subjected to tension from spindle fibres. Later spreading of oocytes, which matured for 6 h, was done to detect precocious chiasma resolution due to attachment of chromosomes to microtubules from opposite spindle poles. Univalents were virtually absent from all oocytes spread and C-banded after 3 h or 6 h of maturation. Instead, about 90% of all oocytes contained at least one or several bivalents with a very distal chiasma. In about 70% of all oocytes from both age groups cultured for 3 h or 6 h, chromosomes with one distal chiasma were present in which telomeres of homologues visibly touched each other. Frequently, there were also bivalents with only one distal chiasma in which homologues were separated by a smaller (<0.8 mm) or larger (0.8–2.4 mm) unstained gap. Achiasmatic chromosomes/true univalents do not exhibit a physical association of their homologues in spread oocytes (as shown for instance in oocytes of recombination deficient mutant *Mhl1* mice; Woods et al. 1999). Therefore, it appears that all chromosomes had at least one exchange. The percentage of oocytes containing one or more bivalent with a gap was significantly higher in the aged population (about 75%) compared to the young population (between 59% and 47% of all oocytes cultured for 3 h or 6 h, respectively; G. Michel et al., manuscript submitted). The percentage of oocytes, which contained bivalents with a gap and the absolute numbers of such presumably susceptible chromosomal configurations, did not increase during culture. From a total of over 2,000 bivalents examined in young oocytes after 3 h and 6 h of culture, 8.7% and 8.6% had a single distal chiasma without a gap, and 5% and 3.8% had one exchange close to the telomere with a gap, respectively. In the aged population of oocytes, of 1,760 and over 2,000 bivalents scored (with spreading at 3 h or 6 h, respectively), 9.6% and 10.8% had a distal chiasma without a gap, and 8.3% and 9% had one exchange close to the telomere with a gap.

In conclusion, there is no increase in univalents with advanced maturation, which may be related to premature detachment of homologues upon bipolar attachment and tension on chromosomes. Also, there is no increase in the percentage of bivalents with a gap, which could be interpreted as detachment of homologues, premature chiasma resolution or predivision at this stage. However, there is a significant correlation between reproductive age, depleted follicle pool, and the numbers of oocytes, which possess chromosomes with one extremely distal exchange resulting in an unstained gap between telomeres on spread chromosomes. The relative percentage of bivalents with a gap and the average numbers of bivalents with distal chiasma, which are in one oocyte, increase with advanced maternal age. There are three explanations for this. (1) A pool of oocytes characterized by a particular pattern of recombination is retained in the ovaries until its near depletion in accordance with the existence of a "production line". (2) Follicles with oocytes that have high numbers of bivalents with a distal chiasma are not induced to transit from the resting to the growing pool at young maternal ages but do so at advanced age, or there is no selection against follicles containing "bad" oocytes with high numbers of potentially risky configurations at advanced reproductive ages. (3) Contact between sister chromatids has been lost during prolonged meiotic arrest in the aged, dictyate stage-arrested oocytes, but telomere cohesion is still maintained in the bivalents. Currently, it is not possible to discriminate between these aetiological factors.

8.6.2 Hormonal Status and Aneuploidy at Metaphase II in Mouse Oocytes

Chromosomal analysis showed that higher numbers of oocytes from aged mice had extra metaphase II chromosomes or single or multiple chromatids at meiosis II as compared to young oocytes, which were obtained from natural cycles, although all oocytes matured under identical conditions in vitro (G. Michel et al., manuscript submitted). Hyperploidy was also higher in aged as compared to young oocytes obtained from the ovaries of mice, which were previously primed with pregnant mare serum (PMS) but the age difference was not significant under these conditions. Aged oocytes possessed significantly more often single or multiple chromatids at metaphase II, irrespective of whether oocytes came from spontaneous or stimulated cycles (G. Michel et al., manuscript submitted). Some of these must have derived by predivision, since single chromatids were found in the oocyte and in the corresponding polar body.

In conclusion, the observations imply that fidelity of chromosome segregation was compromised by reproductive ageing in oocytes of the CBA/Ca mouse. The initiating event and lesions were already fixed in the aged oocytes before maturation. Hormonal homeostasis prior to resumption of maturation modulated susceptibility to errors in chromosome segregation in our model (G. Michel et al., manuscript submitted). Although 90% of the young oocytes contained one or more bivalents with only one distal chiasma, the majority of them were capable of supporting normal chromosome segregation. In contrast, the aged oocytes, which contained potentially susceptible chromosomes, were characterized by frequent errors in chromosome segregation and disturbed timing of separation of chromatids. Global low levels of recombination have been observed in association with trisomy 21 (Brown et al. 2000). This suggests that the chromosomal state as it is derived from early meiotic events as well as other cytoplasmic factors, which control timing at maturation contribute to risks for aneuploidy.

8.6.3 Aberrant Cell Cycle and Activity of Kinases in Aged Oocytes

It appears that in vitro maturation of human oocytes is often slower in the population of GV oocytes obtained from aged as compared to young women (e.g. Angell 1991; Volarcik et al. 1998). Human oocytes of aged women frequently form aberrant spindles and have a significant delay or failure in congression of chromosomes to the spindle equator (Battaglia et al. 1996; Volarcik et al. 1998). Aged oocytes of the mouse appear to enter anaphase I earlier as those from young females (Eichenlaub-Ritter and Boll 1989; G. Michel et al., manuscript submitted). In order to obtain more information on the origin of altered kinetics in meiosis, we analysed the activity of meiotic kinases, which drive the cell cycle or are involved in meiotic arrest in the CBA/Ca mouse model. Aged oocytes tended to go more synchronously and readily to GVBD as compared to young ones (G. Michel et al., manuscript submitted). Also, they reproducibly emitted a polar body (PB) earlier than the young controls. Relative activity of MPF and mitogen-activated protein (MAP) kinases, which are components of cytostatic factor and become activated downstream from the Mos kinase, can be determined in cell extracts from oocytes (e.g. Fulka et al. 1992; Verlhac et al. 1994). From comparison of kinase activity in cell extracts of young and aged oocytes, it appears that the increase in MPF and MAP kinase activity, which occurs after GVBD (3 h of culture), is delayed in aged as compared to young oocytes, although the aged oocytes initiate anaphase I and emit a polar body more readily, synchronously and earlier than the young oocytes (G. Michel et al., manuscript submitted). MAP kinase activity is required for spindle formation (Verlhac et al. 1994) and chromosomes do not properly condense in oocytes, which lack MAP kinase activity (Lu et al. 2002). In conclusion, our observations suggest that there is a asynchrony in cytoplasmic and nuclear maturation events in aged oocytes.

Anaphase in somatic cells is initiated at a cell-type dependent interval after all chromosomes have congressed to the spindle equator (Rieder et al. 1994). In mammalian oocytes, the relative length of maturation before anaphase I appears to depend on the homeostasis, expression and degradation of cyclin B, the regulatory subunit of MPF (Ledan et al. 2001). Our observations indicate that the control of meiotic progression is compromised in aged oocytes, which may relate to differences in turnover of cyclins or other molecules involved in meiotic timing. In fact, Steuerwald et al. (2001) recently reported that the relative abundance of Mad2 mRNA is reduced in human oocytes obtained from aged patients as compared to those from young women. Mad2 protein is one of the proteins in checkpoint control at the anaphase transition (Gardner and Burke 2000). We postulate that ageing affects the expression and regulation of cell cycle-regulating genes, and possibly also of genes, which are controlling monopolar attachment of sister chromatids at meiosis I (e.g. monopolin, Toth et al. 2000). When oocytes are induced to trigger anaphase I when the meiotic window in which checkpoint control is expressed has not been reached or is compromised because of low abundance of checkpoint proteins, they may separate chromosomes randomly when there is congression failure or inappropriate orientation/attachment. Compromised spindle formation in human oocytes may result in a relative delay of the time of checkpoint activation. Similar to the mouse, initiation of anaphase I by critical reduction in availability of cyclin B in aged human oocytes may then also result in progression to anaphase I with unaligned chromosomes. We have previously shown that meiotic delay induced by exposure of mouse oocytes to diazepam is associated with predivision of some chromosomes and displacement of individual chromosomes from the spindle equator (Sun et al. 2001). Susceptibility to predivision was similar for the three mouse chromosomes, which were identified by FISH, while congression failure was chromosome-specific. Differential behaviour of chromosomes in altered cell cycles could explain the chromosome-specific susceptibility to aneuploidy as implied by the trisomy data.

8.7 Cell–Cell Interactions, and Expression and Aneuploidy in Oocytes

It is predominantly during oocyte growth when the female germ cell becomes endowed with rRNA, tRNAs, mRNA and proteins, which are essential for maturation and the early stages of preimplantation development prior to zygotic gene activation (reviewed by Eichenlaub-Ritter and Peschke 2002). For acquisition of full meiotic competence, it is essential that proteins, which regulate cell cycle progression, are accumulated and localized correctly before maturation is resumed (e.g. Mitra and Schultz 1996). Studies in the mouse suggest that oocytes become expressionally repressed transiently prior to the major luteinizing hormone (LH) surge, after a phase of active gene expression during oocyte growth. This depends on efficient signalling between granulosa cells and the oocyte (e.g. De La Fuente and Eppig 2001). Prolonging the repressed state appears to upset control of chromosome segregation in mouse oocytes (Zuccotti et al. 1998). Assuming that depletion of the follicle pool affects the timing during folliculogenesis, a extended arrest of human oocytes with transcriptionally silenced nucleus may initiate apoptosis and predispose the oocyte to aberrant expression of cell cycle-regulating proteins, e.g. those that are involved in spindle formation and cell cycle control in oocytes as well as those required for development of the embryo after fertilization. Early stages of apoptosis have been frequently observed in oocytes from aged women (Wu et al. 2000). Reduced vascularization, which may compromise follicular maturation, could contribute to inappropriate gene expression and reduced oocyte quality (Gaulden 1992; Van Blerkom 2000). Inappropriate hormonal environment at folliculogenesis may result from altered feedback in FSH secretion, inhibin production and subtle differences in the differentiation and interactions of somatic cells and oocytes within the follicle when the follicle pool is depleted (te Velde and Pearson 2002). We have preliminary evidence that culture conditions influence chromatid cohesion in chromosomes of oocytes. Since meiotic and developmental capacity of oocytes directly relates to oocyte-granulosa cell interactions (e.g. Carabatsos et al. 2000) and hormonal homeostasis, it is feasible that inefficient signalling between somatic and germ cells and depletion of the follicle pool may result in high susceptibility to untimely chromosome segregation, similar to what is observed in oocytes maturing in vitro in a suboptimal microenvironment, which we experimentally induced.

8.8 Summary and Future Prospects

The retrospective analysis of the origin and recombinational history of extra chromosomes in human trisomies has suggested that maternal ageing is associated with a high risk for errors in chromosome segregation at first meiotic division of oogenesis. Individual chromosomes appear differentially susceptible to errors in segregation with age. Chromosomal analysis of spare, donated or unfertilized human oocytes and preimplantation embryos suggest that chromosomal imbalance is one major cause of the limited developmental potential of many human conceptuses and low success in assisted reproduction. From trisomy data, it appears that cytoplasmic, oocyte intrinsic factors associated with maternal ageing and the presence of susceptible chromosomes both contribute to aneuploidy and precocious chromatid segregation. Studies in a mouse model imply that cell cycle control is abnormal during resumption of maturation in aged oocytes and that hormonal environment prior to resumption of maturation influences oocyte quality and capacity to segregate chromosomes. We propose that depletion of the follicle pool adversely affects folliculogenesis and oocyte growth and quality with consequences for expression pattern and timing at maturation. In support of this hypothesis, there are reports suggesting that the risk for a trisomic conceptus is related to follicle pool size rather than age of the woman. Also, the expression of critical genes in checkpoint control of anaphase progression appears altered in aged human oocytes. Future studies have to show whether dissociation of meiotic proteins from chromosomes at prophase I in oocytes but not spermatocytes may contribute to the sex-specific high risk for errors in chromosome segregation during meiotic divisions. Prospective studies in experimental animals should be aimed at analysis of aetiological factors in oocyte aneuploidy and identification of culture conditions or treatments, which improve oocyte quality and support high fidelity in chromosome segregation at oogenesis.

Acknowledgements. The expert technical assistance by Ilse Betzendahl and critical reading of the manuscript by Rudolf Eichenlaub are gratefully acknowledged. The work has been supported by EU (QLK4–2000–00058).

References

Angell RR (1991) Predivision in human oocytes at meiosis I, a mechanism for trisomy formation in man. Hum Genet 86:383–387

Angell R (1997) First-meiotic-division nondisjunction in human oocytes. Am J Hum Genet 61:23–32

Battaglia DE, Goodwin P, Klein NA, et al (1996) Influence of maternal age on meiotic spindle assembly in oocytes from naturally cycling women. Mol Hum Reprod 11:2217–2222

Benadiva CA, Kligman I, Munné S (1996) Aneuploidy 16 in human embryos increases significantly with maternal age. Fertil Steril 666:248–255

Benzaken B, Martin-Pont B, Bergere M, et al (1998) Chromosome 21 detection in human oocyte fluorescence in situ hybridization: possible effect of maternal age. J Ass Reprod Genet 15:105–110

Bhal PS, Pugh ND, Gregory L, et al (2001) Perifollicular vascularity as a potential variable affecting outcome in stimulated intrauterine insemination treatment cycles: a study using transvaginal power Doppler. Hum Reprod 16:1682–1689

Bond DJ, Chandley AC (1983) Aneuploidy. Oxford monographs on medical genetics No. 11. Oxford University Press, Oxford

Brook JD, Gosden RG, Chandley AC (1984) Maternal age and aneuploid embryos: evidence from the mouse that biological and not chronological age is the important influence. Hum Genet 6:41–45

Brown AS, Feingold E, Broman KW, et al (2000) Genome-wide variation in recombination in female meiosis: a risk factor for non-disjunction of chromosome 21. Hum Mol Genet 9:515–523

Brunet S, Maria AS, Guillaud P, et al (1999) Kinetochore fibers are not involved in the formation of the first meiotic spindle in mouse oocytes, but control the exit from the first meiotic M phase. J Cell Biol 146:1–12

Buonomo SB, Clyne RK, Fuchs J et al (2000) Disjunction of homologous chromosomes in meiosis I depends on proteolytic cleavage of the meiotic cohesin *Rec8* by separin. Cell 103:387–398

Bugge M, Collins A, Peterson M, et al (1998) Non-disjunction of chromosome 18. Hum Mol Genet 7:661–669

Caligara C, Navarro J, Vargas G et al (2001) The effect of repeated controlled ovarian stimulation in donors. Hum Reprod 16:2320–2323

Carabatsos MJ, Sellitto C, Goodenough DA, et al (2000) Oocyte-granulosa cell heterologous gap junctions are required for the coordination of nuclear and cytoplasmic meiotic competence. Dev Biol 226:167–179

Clyde JM, Gosden RG, Rutherford AJ, et al (2001) Demonstration of a mechanism of aneuploidy in human oocytes using Multifluor fluorescence in situ hybridization. Fertil Steril 76:837–840

Coulam CB, Goodman C, Rinehart JS (1999) Colour Doppler indices of follicular blood flow as predictors of pregnancy after in-vitro fertilization and embryo transfer. Hum Reprod 14:1979–1982

Crowley PH, Gulati DK, Hayden TL, et al (1979) A chiasma-hormonal hypothesis relating Down's syndrome and maternal age. Nature 280:417–418

Dailey T, Dale B, Cohen J, et al (1996) Association between nondisjunction and maternal age in meiosis-II human oocytes. Am J Hum Genet 59:176–184

De La Fuente R, Eppig JJ (2001) Transcriptional activity of the mouse oocyte genome: companion granulosa cells modulate transcription and chromatin remodeling. Dev Biol 229:224–236

Delhanty JD, Harper JC, Ao A, et al (1997) Multicolour FISH detects frequent chromosomal mosaicism and chaotic division in normal preimplantation embryos from fertile patients. Hum Genet 99:755–760

Eichenlaub-Ritter U (1996) Parental age-related aneuploidy in human germ cells and offspring: a story of past and present. Environ Mol Mutagen 28:211–236

Eichenlaub-Ritter U (1998) Genetics of oocyte ageing. Maturitas 30:143–169

Eichenlaub-Ritter U (2000) The determinants of non-disjunction and their possible relationship with oocyte ageing. In: te Velde ER, Pearson PL, Broekmans FJ (eds) Studies in profertility series 9: female reproductive aging. Parthenon, New York, pp 149–184

Eichenlaub-Ritter U, Boll I (1989) Nocodazole sensitivity, age-related aneuploidy, and alterations in the cell cycle during maturation of mouse oocytes. Cytogenet Cell Genet 52:170–176

Eichenlaub-Ritter U, Peschke M (2002) Expression in in vivo and in vitro growing and maturing oocytes: focus on regulation of expression at the translational level. Hum Reprod Update (in press)

Eichenlaub-Ritter U, Chandley AC, Gosden RG (1988) The CBA mouse as a model for age-related aneuploidy in man: studies of oocyte maturation, spindle formation and chromosome alignment during meiosis. Chromosoma 96:220–226

Fabricant JD, Schneider E (1978) Studies on the genetic and immunologic components of the maternal age effect. Dev Biol 66:41–45

Faddy MJ (2000) Follicle dynamics during ovarian ageing. Mol Cell Endocrinol 163:43–48

Freeman SB, Yang Q, Allran K (2000) Women with a reduced ovarian complement may have an increased risk for a child with Down syndrome. Am J Hum Genet 66:1680–1683

Fritz B, Hallermann C, Olert J, et al (2001) Cytogenetic analyses of culture failures by comparative genomic hybridisation (CGH)-Re-evaluation of chromosome aberration rates in early spontaneous abortions. Eur J Hum Genet 9:539–547

Fulka J Jr, Jung T, Moor RM (1992) The fall of biological maturation promoting factor (MPF) and histone H1 kinase activity during anaphase and telophase in mouse oocytes. Mol Reprod Dev 32:378–382

Gardner RD, Burke DJ (2000) The spindle checkpoint: two transitions, two pathways. Trends Cell Biol 10:154–218

Gaulden ME (1992) Maternal age-effect: the enigma of Down syndrome and other trisomic conditions. Mutation Res 296:69–88

Gianaroli L, Magli MC, Ferraretti AP, et al (1999) Preimplantation diagnosis for aneuploidies in patients undergoing in vitro fertilization with a poor prognosis: identification of the categories for which it should be proposed. Fertil Steril 72:837–844

Gosden RG (1973) Chromosome anomalies of preimplantation mouse embryos in relation to maternal age. J Reprod Fertil 35:351–354

Gras L, McBain J, Trounson A, et al (1992) The incidence of chromosomal aneuploidy in stimulated and unstimulated [natural] uninseminated human oocytes. Hum Reprod 7:1396–1401

Harrison RH, Kuo HC, Scriven PN (2000) Lack of cell cycle checkpoints in human cleavage stage embryos revealed by a clonal pattern of chromosomal mosaicism analysed by sequential multicolour FISH. Zygote 8:217–224

Hassold TJ (1998) Nondisjunction in the human male. Curr Topics Dev Biol 37:383–406

Hassold T, Hunt P (2001) To err (meiotically) is human: the genesis of human aneuploidy. Nat Rev Genet 2:280–291

Hassold TJ, Sherman SL, Pettay D, et al (1991) XY chromosome nondisjunction in man is associated with diminished recombination in the pseudoautosomal region. Am J Hum Genet 49:253–260

Hassold TJ, Merrill M, Adkins K, et al (1995) Recombination and maternal age-related non-disjunction: molecular studies of trisomy 16. Am J Hum Genet 57:867–874

Hassold T, Sherman S, Hunt P (2000) Counting cross-overs: characterizing meiotic recombination in mammals. Hum Mol Genet 9:2409–2419

Henderson SA, Edwards RG (1968) Chiasma frequency and maternal age in mammals. Nature 217:22–28

Hodges CA, LeMaire-Adkins R, Hunt PA (2001) Coordinating the segregation of sister chromatids during the first meiotic division: evidence for sexual dimorphism. J Cell Sci 114:2417–2426

Iwarsson E, Lundqvist M, Inzunza J, et al (1999) A high degree of aneuploidy in frozen-thawed human preimplantation embryos. Hum Genet 104:376–382

Jamieson ME, Coutts JR, Connor JM (1994) The chromosome constitution of human preimplantation embryos fertilized in vitro. Mol Hum Reprod 9:709–715

Keefe DL, Niven-Fairchild T, Powell S, et al (1995) Mitochondrial deoxyribonucleic acid deletions in oocytes and reproductive aging in women. Fertil Steril 64:577–583

Kline J, Kinney A, Levin B, et al (2000) Trisomic pregnancy and earlier age at menopause. Am J Hum Genet 67:395–404

Koehler KE, Hawley RS, Sherman S, et al (1996) Recombination and nondisjunction in humans and flies. Hum Mol Genet 5:1495–1504

Lamb NE, Freeman SB, Savage-Austin A, et al (1996) Susceptible chiasmate configurations of chromosome 21 predispose to non-disjunction in both maternal meiosis I and meiosis II. Nat Genet 14:400–405

Lamb NE, Feingold E, Savage A, et al (1997) Characterization of susceptible chiasma configurations that increase the risk for maternal nondisjunction of chromosome 21. Hum Mol Genet 6:1391–1399

Ledan E, Polanski Z, Terret ME (2001) Meiotic maturation of the mouse oocyte requires an equilibrium between cyclin B synthesis and degradation. Dev Biol 232:400–413

Lee JY, Orr-Weaver TL (2001) The molecular basis of sister-chromatid cohesion. Annu Rev Cell Dev Biol 17:753–777

LeMaire-Adkins E, Radke K, Hunt PA (1997) Lack of checkpoint control at the metaphase-anaphase transition: a mechanism of meiotic non-disjunction in mammalian females. J Cell Biol 139:1611–1619

LeMaire-Adkins R, Hunt PA (2000) Nonrandom segregation of the mouse univalent X chromosome: evidence of spindle-mediated meiotic drive. Genetics 156:775–783

Libby BJ, De La Fuente R, O'Brien MJ, et al (2002) The mouse meiotic mutation mei1 disrupts chromosome synapsis with sexually dimorphic consequences for meiotic progression. Dev Biol 242:174–187

Lu Q, Dunn RL, Angeles R, et al (2002) Regulation of spindle formation by active mitogen-activated protein kinase and protein phosphatase 2 a during mouse oocyte meiosis. Biol Reprod 66:29–37

MacDonald M, Hassold TJ, Harvey J (1994) The origin of 47,XXY and 47,XXX aneuploidy: heterogeneous mechanisms and role of aberrant recombination. Hum Mol Genet 3:1365–1371

Mahmood R, Brierley CH, Faed MJ, et al (2000) Mechanisms of maternal aneuploidy: FISH analysis of oocytes and polar bodies in patients undergoing assisted conception. Hum Genet 106:620–626

Mailhes JB, Young D, London SN (1998) Postovulatory ageing of mouse oocytes in vivo and premature centromere separation and aneuploidy. Biol Reprod 58:1206–1210

Márquez C, Cohen J, Munné S (1998) Chromosome identification in human oocytes and polar bodies by spectral karyotyping. Cytogenet Cell Genet 81:254–258

Márquez C, Sandalinas M, Bahçe M, et al (2000) Chromosome abnormalities in 1255 cleavage-stage human embryos. Reprod Biomed Online 1:17–27

Martini E, Flaherty SP, Swann NJ (2000) FISH analysis of six chromosomes in unfertilized human oocytes after polar body removal. J Assist Reprod Genet 17:276–283

Mitra J, Schultz RM (1996) Regulation of the acquisition of meiotic competence in the mouse: changes in the subcellular localization of cdc2, cyclin B1, cdc25 C and wee1, and in the concentration of these proteins and their transcripts. J Cell Sci 109:2407–2415

Muller-Hocker J, Schafer S, Weis S, et al (1996) Morphological-cytochemical and molecular genetic analyses of mitochondria in isolated human oocytes in the reproductive age. Mol Hum Reprod 2:951–958

Munné S, Cohen J (1998) Chromosome abnormalities in human embryos. Hum Reprod Update 4:842–855

Nakaoka Y, Okamoto E, Miharu N. et al (1998) Chromosome analysis in human oocytes remaining unfertilized after in-vitro insemination: effect of maternal age and fertilization rate. Hum Reprod 13:419–424

Nasmyth K (2001) Disseminating the genome: joining, resolving, and separating sister chromatids during mitosis and meiosis. Annu Rev Genet 35:673–745

Nicklas RB, Waters JC, Salmon ED, et al (2001) Checkpoint signals in grasshopper meiosis are sensitive to microtubule attachment, but tension is still essential. J Cell Sci 114:4173–4183

Parisi S, McKay MJ, Molnar M, et al (1999) Rec8p, a meiotic recombination and sister chromatid cohesion phosphoprotein of the Rad21p family is conserved from fission yeast to humans. Mol Cell Biol 19:3515–3528

Penrose LS (1933) The relative effects of paternal and maternal age in mongolism. J Genet 27:219–224

Plachot M (2001) Chromosomal abnormalities in oocytes. Mol Cell Endocrinol 183(Suppl 1):S59–S63

Polani PE, Crolla JA (1981) A test of the production line hypothesis of mammalian oogenesis. Hum Genet 88:64–70

Rieder CL, Schultz A, Cole R, et al (1994) Anaphase onset in vertebrate somatic cells is controlled by a checkpoint that monitors sister kinetochore attachment to the spindle. J Cell Biol 127:1301–1310

Robinson WP, Kuchinka, B., Bernasconi F, et al (1998) Maternal meiosis I non-disjunction of chromosome 15: dependence of the maternal age effect on level of recombination. Hum Mol Genet 7:1011–1019

Roeder GS, Bailis JM (2000) The pachytene checkpoint. Trends Genet 16:395–403

Sakurada K, Ishikawa H, Endo A (1996) Cytogenetic effects of advanced maternal age and delayed fertilization on first-cleavage mouse embryos. Cytogenet Cell Genet 72:46–49

Schon EA, Kim SH, Ferreira JC, et al (2000) Chromosomal non-disjunction in human oocytes: is there a mitochondrial connection? Hum Reprod 15(Suppl 2):160–172

Sears DD, Hegemann JH, Hieter P (1992) Meiotic recombination and segregation of human-derived artificial chromosomes in Saccharomyces cerevisiae. Proc Natl Acad Sci USA 89:5296–5300

Shonn MA, McCarroll R, Murray AW (2000) Requirement of the spindle checkpoint for proper chromosome segregation in budding yeast meiosis. Science 289:300–303

Soewarto D, Schmiady H, Eichenlaub-Ritter U (1995) Consequences of non-extrusion of the first polar body and control of the sequential segregation of homologues and chromatids in mammalian oocytes. Hum Reprod 10:2350–2360

Steuerwald N, Cohen J, Herrera RJ, et al (2001) Association between spindle assembly checkpoint expression and maternal age in human oocytes. Mol Hum Reprod 7:49–55

Sudakin V, Chan GK, Yen TJ (2001) Checkpoint inhibition of the APC/C in HeLa cells is mediated by a complex of BUBR1, BUB3, CDC20, and MAD2. J Cell Biol 154:925–936

Sugawara S, Mikamo K (1983) Absence of correlation between univalent formation and meiotic nondisjunction in aged female Chinese hamsters. Cytogenet Cell Genet 35:34–40

Sun F, Yin H, Eichenlaub-Ritter U (2001) Differential chromosome behaviour in mammalian oocytes exposed to the tranquilizer diazepam in vitro. Mutagenesis 16:407–417

Tarin JJ (1996) Potential effects of age-associated oxidative stress on mammalian oocytes/embryos. Mol Hum Reprod 2:717–724

Tay J, Richter JD (2001) Germ cell differentiation and synaptonemal complex formation are disrupted in CPEB knockout mice. Dev Cell 1:201–213 te Velde E, Pearson P (2002) The variability of female reproductive ageing. Hum Reprod Update 8:141–154

Toth A, Rabitsch KP, Galova M (2000) Functional genomics identifies monopolin: a kinetochore protein required for segregation of homologs during meiosis I. Cell 103:1155–1168

Van Blerkom J (2000) Intrafollicular influences on human oocyte developmental competence: perifollicular vascularity, oocyte metabolism and mitochondrial function. Hum Reprod 15(Suppl 2):173–188

Van Blerkom J, Davis P (2001) Differential effects of repeated ovarian stimulation on cytoplasmic and spindle organization in metaphase II mouse oocytes matured in vivo and in vitro. Mol Hum Reprod 16:757–764

Vaskivuo TE, Anttonen M, Herva R, et al (2001) Survival of human ovarian follicles from fetal to adult life: apoptosis, apoptosis-related proteins, and transcription factor GATA-4.Clin Endocrinol Metab 86:3421–3429.

Verlhac MH, Kubiak J, Clarke HJ, et al (1994) Microtubule and chromatin behaviour follow MAP kinase activity but not MPF during meiosis in mouse oocytes. Development 120:1017–1025

Verlinsky Y, Cieslak J, Ivakhnenko V, et al (2001) Chromosomal abnormalities in the first and second polar body. Mol Cell Endocrinol 183(Suppl 1):S47–S49

Volarcik K, Sheean L, Goldfarb J, et al (1998) The meiotic competence of human oocytes is influenced by donor age: evidence that folliculogenesis is compromised in the reproductively aged ovary. Hum Reprod 13:154–160

Warburton D, Kinney A (1996) Chromosomal differences in suceptibility to meiotic aneuploidy. Environ Mol Mutagen 28:237–247

Wells D, Delhanty JD (2000) Comprehensive chromosomal analysis of human preimplantation embryos using whole genome amplification and single cell comparative genomic hybridization. Mol Hum Reprod 6:1055–1062

Wilding M, Dale B, Marino M, et al (2001) Mitochondrial aggregation patterns and activity in human oocytes and preimplantation embryos. Hum Reprod 16:909–917

Wolstenholme J, Angell RR (2000) Maternal age and trisomy – a unifying mechanism of formation. Chromosoma 109:435–438

Woods LM, Hodges CA, Baart E, et al (1999) Chromosomal influence on meiotic spindle assembly: abnormal meiosis I in female Mlh1 mutant mice. J Cell Biol 145:1395–1406

Wu J, Zhang L, Wang X (2000) Maturation and apoptosis of human oocytes in vitro are age-related. Fertil Steril 74:1137–1141

Zuccotti M, Boiani M, Garagna S (1998) Analysis of aneuploidy rate in antral and ovulated mouse oocytes during female aging. Mol Reprod Dev 50:305–331

9 Ovarian Infertility – Reasons and Treatment Paradigms

M. Ludwig, K. Diedrich

9.1 Introduction 137
9.2 Post-surgical Ovarian Infertility 138
9.3 Primary Ovarian Failure 139
9.4 Non-surgical Destruction of Ovarian Function 139
9.5 Premature Ovarian Failure 141
9.6 Clinical Work-up of a Patient with Premature Ovarian Failure . . . 146
9.7 Treatment Options in Cases of Premature Ovarian Failure 148
9.8 Alternative Treatment Options 150
9.9 Conclusion 153
References 154

9.1 Introduction

Infertility is defined as the inability to conceive a child after one to two years of regular unprotected sexual intercourse. Interestingly, the prevalence of infertility has not changed over the past 100 years. Reports from Australia a century ago show a prevalence of about 12% women who cannot conceive, and this is still true for industrialized countries (Snick et al. 1997).

Other statistics have shown that the distribution of causes for infertility is equally distributed to the male and female partner. In the female partner, ovulatory dysfunction is the most prevalent cause. However, pure ovarian dysfunction is rare. Mostly, other systems are also involved. The most common endocrine disorder is the polycystic ovarian syndrome (PCOS), a hypothalamic-pituitary-ovarian dysregulation. Even if ovarian problems are also involved with PCOS, the condition is more than pure ovarian infertility.

Ovarian infertility is a disorder in which the woman is not able to produce fertilizable oocytes due to problems which primarily involve the ovaries themselves. This is the case when either:

- The ovaries have been surgically removed in the past
- Ovarian reproductive function has never started
- Ovarian function has been destroyed by radio- or chemotherapy especially in cases of childhood cancer
- Ovarian function has started, but stopped before the 40th year of life – so-called premature ovarian failure (POF)

For a better understanding of the different subgroups we have subdivided this chapter into these four different conditions, even if all of them belong – in a wider sense – to the term "premature ovarian failure".

9.2 Post-surgical Ovarian Infertility

Different situations are possible, which can lead to a removal of ovaries. These are, for example, severe tuboovarian abscesses, which cannot be managed conservatively by drainage and i.v. antibiotics, recurrent ovarian cysts, which have been removed due to clinical symptoms in the patient, severe endometriosis, ovarian tumors like teratoma, or even ovarian carcinoma early in life.

Patients' histories, where parts of the ovary or even a total ovary have been removed due to ovarian tumors or cysts, and where subsequently a similar problem occurs on the contralateral side, are seen regularly in clinical practice.

This has lead to a more careful decision making for surgical intervention in those cases, for the trial with hormonal therapies in cases of functional cysts, and, overall, to a much more conservative way of treatment.

However, in case that ovaries have been removed bilaterally, only oocyte donation can help a woman to become pregnant herself – as long as she still has a functional uterus and endometrium. Otherwise, treatment options could include surrogate motherhood and counseling the couple about the possibility of adoption.

9.3 Primary Ovarian Failure

Primary ovarian failure leads to primary amenorrhea – defined as the menarche, which has not been started at 16 years of age. Possible causes are, for example, chromosomal aberrations, anatomic malformations of the inner genital tract, or endocrine abnormalities. Treatment options in these cases are quite the same as those in cases of post-surgical ovarian infertility.

9.4 Non-surgical Destruction of Ovarian Function

In cases of childhood cancer, high dose chemotherapies and/or radiotherapies offer a good chance for a disease-free survival of the child. As the survival rate of children with malignancies has increased over the past few decades, these children nowadays not rarely reach adulthood. In young adulthood too, leukemias and lymphomas can be cured by these therapeutic approaches. However, different chemotherapeutics have proven to have direct ovarian toxicity – even if a certain threshold toxicity dose of the single medication is not known in most cases. This is difficult to assess, since most chemotherapeutics are used in combinations, and therefore the combinatory effect – more than the single agent alone – leads to destruction of ovarian function. The dose for sterilization is 600 cGy, even if in single cases even higher doses to the pelvis have been administered without reducing ovarian function (Anasti 1998). Especially in cases of lymphomas that involved lymph nodes in the abdominal cavity, radiotherapy is a common approach and might lead to subsequent problems with reproductive function in adulthood.

Prevention of these deleterious effects has been discussed in the literature. A promising approach is ovarian protection by surgical intervention and laparoscopic oophoropexy, i.e., transposition of the ovaries out of the radiation field (Williams et al. 1999). This can avoid irradiation damage.

In cases of chemotherapy, it might be helpful to prevent ovarian damage by stopping ovarian function. This approach has been discussed, since it is well known, that prepubertal children are more protected against chemotherapeutic agents than are postpubertal children. To do this, either a contraceptive pill, or, more recently, gonadotropin-releasing hormone (GnRH) analogies have been chosen. Prospective, randomized studies do not exist to date. The largest prospective, historically controlled series has been published by Blumenfeld et al. They administered a GnRH agonist prior to chemotherapy for Hodgkin's or non-Hodgkin's disease in more than 50 patients. Compared to a historical control group, there was only 4% of disturbed ovarian function in the study, but 60% in the control group (Blumenfeld et al. 1996, 1997; Blumenfeld and Avivi 1999).

Therefore, despite limited experience and the lack of prospective, randomized data in the literature, the administration of GnRH analogues should be offered to each woman who undergoes chemotherapy – especially after puberty.

Since in these cases the chemotherapy is commonly started within a few days, a combined use of GnRH agonists and antagonists should be chosen. GnRH agonists will result first in a flare-up effect with a pituitary release of luteinizing hormone (LH) and follicle-stimulating hormone (FSH) and then in ovarian stimulation – which should be avoid in case of a chemotherapy. Pituitary suppression is achieved after 10–14 days. GnRH antagonists, on the other hand, will lead to pituitary suppression within 3–6 h, have no flare-up effect – but are until now not available as a depot preparation. Therefore, it is suitable and most comfortable for the patient to administer 3 mg of the GnRH antagonist cetrorelix (Cetrotide 3 mg, Serono International S.A., Geneva, Switzerland) every 3–5 days and to start the administration of a GnRH agonist depot preparation in a 4-week interval in the first pause between two chemotherapies, which should be at least 10–14 days long. The exact interval of cetrorelix administration can be triggered by serum estradiol levels, which should not exceed a maximum of 50 pg/ml. However, to be on the safe side, a 4-day interval should be the easiest and most practical approach.

In parallel to such a therapy, an oral contraceptive pill or a preparation for hormonal replacement therapy can be administered to prevent hormonal withdrawal symptoms and long-term sequelae of sexual steroid depletion like osteoporosis. This, of course, is not indicated in cases of hormonal sensitive tumors.

When patients have survived childhood cancer after treatment, a damage to the oocytes in the sense of a higher rate of malformations in subsequently born children seems not have to be expected.

9.5 Premature Ovarian Failure

9.5.1 Risk of Premature Ovarian Failure

In contrast to the other clinical entities, POF is, in its strict definition, an ovarian-immanent disease, without iatrogenic intervention – when post-surgical and chemotherapy-/radiotherapy-induced cases are excluded. In the wider sense, however, these possibilities also are included under this condition and discussed in the literature together with the following, other causes of POF.

The prevalence of POF is estimated to be 1% of women in their reproductive years (Coulam et al. 1986). Coulam et al. have studied a cohort of 1,858 women born between 1928 and 1932. These were identified in 1950 as residents of Rochester, Minnesota. They showed a prevalence of POF in 0.1% up to 30 years of age, and of 1% up to 40 years of age. The annual incidence of natural menopause per 100,000 person years were 10, 76, and 881, for the ages 15–29, 30–39, and 40–44, respectively.

Furthermore, the diagnosis of POF can be made in 10%–28% of patients with primary amenorrhea, and 4%–18% in patients with secondary amenorrhea (Anasti 1998).

The clinical picture of POF, however, is not limited to ovarian failure but also involves other organ systems. Furthermore, different genetic causes have been discussed, which might be important for a diagnostic work-up. Finally, special treatment options have been considered in cases of POF – in addition to those that are common to all cases of ovarian failure.

Table 1. Inheritance of premature ovarian failure. Data from families (according to Vegetti et al. 1998)

	Total	Sporadic	Familial	*p*
Number of patients (%)	71	49 (69.0)	22 (31.0)	
Median (range) age at premature ovarian failure onset (years)	34 (13–40)	31 (13–40)	37.5 (20–40)	<0.05
Median (range) age of maternal menopause (years)	48 (25–55)	49 (41–55)	40 (25–55)	<0.005

9.5.2 Causes of Premature Ovarian Failure

Principally, the causes can be divided into two categories: patients with follicle depletion and patients with follicle dysfunction. With these two main groups, several subgroups can then be defined (Anasti 1998).

A genetic influence in cases of otherwise non-explainable POF seems to be common. In a multicentric study, Vegetti et al. have examined the genetic history of 71 women with hypergonadotrophic secondary amenorrhea. Patients with known causes of amenorrhea (e.g., postsurgically) or autoimmune disease, as well as those with an abnormal karyotype (e.g., Robertsonian translocations) were excluded. The authors could identify 71 subjects, from which a familial POF was found in 31%. From the pedigree analysis, the authors proposed either a X-linked or autosomal sex-limited inheritance pattern with incomplete penetrance (approx. 80%). The gene could be inherited from the father as well as from the mothers line (Vegetti et al. 1998). More data are shown in the tables (Table 1).

Others have described a familial pattern in 4% (Conway et al. 1996), 12.7% (van Kasteren et al. 1999b), and 22.2% (van Kasteren et al. 1999a).

The prevalence of cytogenetic abnormalities in patients with secondary amenorrhea and POF was found to be about 2.5% (2/79) in a prospective study (Davison et al. 1998). Besides women with 45,X karyotype (Turner's syndrome), also women with 47,XXX karyotype may develop POF (Smith et al. 1974; Villanueva and Rebar 1983). The difference, however, is that Turner's syndrome patients will normally suffer from primary amenorrhea, but triple X syndrome patients will

Table 2. Genes and gene loci involved in the development of premature ovarian failure

Gene/gene locus	Reference	Age at onset of POF	Reference
POF1 (Xq26-qter)	Tharapel et al. 1993 Davison et al. 1998	24–39	Krauss 1987; Tharapel et al. 1993
POF2 (Xq13.3 – Xq21.1)	Powell et al. 1994	16–21	Powell et al. 1994
FMR1 (fragile X premutation) (Xq27.3)	Allingham-Hawking 1999; Uzielli et al. 1999; Conway 1998		
FSH receptor gene	Aittomaki et al. 1996		
INHα (2q33-qter)	Shelling et al. 2000		
deletion Xq26.1	Davison et al. 1998	28–34	Davison et al. 1998
BPES type I (3q22-q23)	Amati 1996		

BPES, blepharophimosis–ptosis–epicanthus inversus syndrome.

have secondary amenorrhea – if at all. Others have studied the prevalence of 45,X/46,XX mosaicism (Devi et al. 1998). They described a significantly higher mean number of X-monosomic cells in a fluorescent in situ hybridization (FISH) analysis in POF patients (n=15) (5.50±1.73), as compared to age-matched controls (n=20) (2.42±1.06), and older women with normal reproductive history (n=10) (3.55±0.73). Therefore, patients with such a mosaicism could have a substantial risk for POF in later life.

With regard to the exact genetic background, different genes or gene loci have been identified, which are involved in certain families in the development of POF. These are shown Table 2.

By X chromosome breakpoint analysis in patients with X-autosome balanced translocations, Sala et al. identified genes in Xq21, which they assumed to be involved in ovarian development (Sala et al. 1997).

The fragile X premutation, at the FMR1 gene at Xq27.3, will lead to POF in 13%–25% of cases (Allingham-Hawkins et al. 1999; Uzielli et al. 1999); on the other hand, 3%–15% of women with POF will be found to have fragile X premutations (Conway et al. 1995; Uzielli et al. 1999; Marozzi et al. 2000). Analyzing the mode of inheritance with fragile X premutations, Hundscheid et al. have proposed a parent-of-origin effect, since they could show that in 28% of individuals with paternally inherited fragile X premutations, but only in 3% of maternally inherited premutations, POF was found. This would have important meanings for counseling patients with fragile X premutations (Hundscheid et al.

2000). This could, however, not be confirmed by others (Murray et al. 2000; Vianna-Morgante and Costa 2000), and was supposed by these authors to be due to an ethnic effect in a defined Dutch population. However, methodological aspects also might have contributed to the divergent results, especially a smaller cohort of patients and/or another risk cohort. An imprinting effect, therefore, is still possible (Sherman 2000).

The FSH receptor gene was described to be defected in certain, single cases of POF (Aittomaki et al. 1996; Beau et al. 1998; Touraine et al. 1999). The C566T mutation was found to be quite common in Finish families, but these or other gene mutations could not be found in other ethnic groups like, for example, Japanese (Takakura et al. 2001), Brazilians (Fonte Kohek et al. 1998), Singapore women (Whitney et al. 1995; Tong et al. 2001), and U.S. citizens (Whitney et al. 1995).

Regarding the action of LH, a recent study showed a higher rate of a certain variant of the LH β-subunit in Japanese women (Takebayashi et al. 2000). In their study, the authors included 245 women with endocrine disorders or gynecologic diseases and 153 healthy control subjects. Within the study population, 15 women with POF were present also, showing significantly more LH variants (53.3%) compared to the controls (8.5%).

In the inhibin gene, a point mutation was identified in 3 out of 43 subjects with POF (7%), but in only 1 out of 150 healthy controls (0.7%). Since this point mutation might lead to an inhibition of receptor binding, it might be involved in the pathogenesis of POF in these cases (Shelling et al. 2000).

Galactosemia also is a condition associated with POF. Here, the development of POF seems to be associated with a special genotype (Q188R/Q188R). Furthermore, certain laboratory markers help to identify high-risk patients within this condition like erythrocyte galactose-1-phosphate level, as well as the recovery of $^{13}CO_2$ from whole body ^{13}C-galactose oxidation (Guerrero et al. 2000). Galactosemia seems to have a direct toxic effect on the ovarian function.

In a substantial subset of patients, different endocrine disorders may be associated with POF – all of them having an autoimmune pathogenesis. These include Hashimoto thyroiditis, Grave's disease, Addison's disease, and diabetes mellitus. Vitiligo, an autoimmune disorder with anti-melanocyte antibodies, is also found in association with POF, as is myasthenia gravis (Kuki et al. 1981).

Alper and Garnet (1985), in a series of 33 patients, reported autoimmune diseases in 18%, including Hashimoto thyroiditis, Grave's disease and vitiligo (Alper and Garner 1985). Ruehsen et al. confirmed these data in a series of 29 patients with 16 having associated autoimmune diseases like Addison's disease, hypothyroidism, or other thyroid diseases (de Moraes et al. 1972). Van Kasteren et al. (1999a) described autoantibodies of different types in 19/36 patients (53%) in a prospective study.

Betterle et al. identified Addison's disease in 18% of their patients (9/50) (Betterle et al. 1993). In a further 20%, other autoimmune diseases could be found, and in 62% of cases no associated autoimmune diseases could be identified in the patients suffering from POF. In another series, the prevalence of Addison's disease was much smaller (3/119, 2.5%) (Kim et al. 1997). The other way around shows that 23% of patients with Addison's disease will develop POF (Turkington and Lebovitz 1967). Others described this risk with 8% in a series of 77 women (Irvine et al. 1968). Since POF normally will precede adrenal failure by several years, subsequent control of adrenal function after diagnosis of POF is of clinical importance (Turkington and Lebovitz 1967; Vazquez and Kenny 1973).

Diabetes mellitus type I occurred in 2.5% in a series of 113 screened patients (Kim et al. 1997). This fits to the prevalence of pancreatic islet-cell antibodies in patients with POF (Belvisi et al. 1993).

Circulating autoimmune ovarian antibodies were described in 59% of patients with otherwise unexplained POF, which was higher compared to different control groups without any disease, or other autoimmune conditions like Grave's disease (Fenichel et al. 1997). The problems of ovarian autoantibodies is that they also can be found non-specifically after surgery (Luborsky et al. 1990), and following oocyte pick-up in an in vitro fertilization cycle (Gobert et al. 1990). Therefore, the real significance of these autoantibodies is difficult to assess.

A special steroid cell autoantibody was identified against 3β-hydroxysteroid dehydrogenase in 21% of patients (Arif et al. 1996). Beside that, however, other autoantibodies against other steroid enzymes, GnRH receptor, etc., have been described to cause oophoritis and subsequent POF.

Rarely, hypoparathyroidism was described to be associated with POF (Golonka and Goodman 1968). Since, however, calcium levels in most patients are normal, this seems to be a rare event.

To conclude, besides certain genetic abnormalities, gene mutations, or specific genetic disorders, autoimmune conditions seem to play a major role in the development of POF. All these things, therefore, have to be taken in account, when a patient with POF is seen in clinical practice.

9.6 Clinical Work-up of a Patient with Premature Ovarian Failure

The clinical work-up must initially include a detailed anamnesis of the patient and her family. This may help to identify other family members suffering from POF, other autoimmune conditions, and consequences for the patient's siblings. It is, for example, well known that in oocyte donation programs, the use of oocytes from a POF patient's sister leads to less good results (Sung et al. 1997), indicating additional genetic factors. In cases of familial POF, siblings should be counseled not to plan conception too late in life.

A physical examination should include a gynecologic work-up and should look for signs of other autoimmune diseases, e.g., vitiligo.

Laboratory screening must include an oral glucose tolerance test, basal thyroid-stimulating hormone (TSH) measurement, an adrenocorticotropic hormone (ACTH) challenge test, and measurement of blood calcium and electrolyte levels. Measurement of antibodies may help to identify patients at risk for other autoimmune diseases in the future. However, these antibodies seem to have no prognostic value for the further development of POF.

Ultrasound will often reveal follicle structures in the ovary. This, however, will not mean that these patients have a higher chance of conceiving in the future. More importantly, three to four measurements of FSH and estradiol levels, with intervals of several weeks, showing postmenopausal levels, will make the final diagnosis of POF.

Ovarian biopsy is the only way to prove whether follicles are still present in the ovary (Olivar 1996). However, ovarian biopsy and subsequent histology have no prognostic value and therefore should not

Table 3. Bone mineral density measurement in patients suffering from premature ovarian failure and a control group (data according to Anasti et al. 1998)

Skeletal site	Number of women (%)		
	≤1SD	≤2SD	≤3SD
Femur neck			
Women with POF (*n*=89)	60 (67)*	17 (19)	2 (2)
Reference group (*n*=218)	35 (16)	6 (2.5)	1 (0.45)
Spine (L2–4)			
Women with POF (*n*=89)	30 (34)*	8 (9)	1 (1)
Reference group (*n*=218)	35 (16)	6 (2.5)	1 (0.45)

POF, premature ovarian failure; SD, standard deviation.
*Significantly different to the reference group ($p<0.001$).

routinely be performed. Only in cases of Y-chromosome material, ovariectomy must be discussed with the patients due to the risk of gonadoblastomas.

After the initial diagnosis, patients must also be counseled about the long-term prognosis of their disease. Physicians must be aware that the diagnosis of POF means an unexpected and severe change in patients' life-planning. Therefore, several counseling sessions should be arranged to help the patient understand the diagnosis, the necessity of subsequent evaluations regarding the development of autoimmune diseases (e.g., Addison's disease, diabetes mellitus), and hormone replacement therapy.

Hormone replacement therapy is important in patients suffering from POF. This, on the one hand, is to avoid short-time sequelae, but also to prevent long-term problems. Anasti et al. could show that even 1.5 years after the cessation of ovarian function due to POF, in 47% of cases femoral neck bone mineral density was more than 1 standard deviation below the mean for a control group ($p<0.01$) (Anasti et al. 1998). More data of this study are shown in Table 3.

Spontaneous pregnancies have been described in several case reports so far (e.g., Check et al. 1989; Menashe et al. 1996; Sheu et al. 1996; Chen and Chang 1997), sometimes after several trials using different ovarian stimulation regimens or oocyte donation. The chance of spontaneous pregnancies is estimated to be about 5%. Therefore, patients should be counseled about this possibility: not to give them the (false) hope of having their own children, but to avoid unwanted pregnancies and subsequent pregnancy termination.

On the other hand, it is important to counsel about the fact that, until now, there has been no proven treatment for these patients – despite many protocols which have been tested. Therefore, counseling should include the possibility of adoption, oocyte donation, and – if indicated – the possibility of surrogate motherhood.

9.7 Treatment Options in Cases of Premature Ovarian Failure

As outlined above, there is no treatment option with a proven efficacy available for these patients. This was also shown in a recent review (van Kasteren and Schoemaker 1999).

Letterie et al. have tried combinations of GnRH agonists and HMG, but did not see any positive effect (Letterie and Miyazawa 1989). Others have tried therapeutic regimens with estrogen or estrogen/progestin combination with the idea to sensitize ovaries to subsequent gonadotrophin stimulation (Lutjen et al. 1986; Check et al. 1989; Tang and Sawers 1989; Gucer et al. 1997), with some pregnancies in single cases (Ohsawa et al. 1985; Leeton et al. 1989; Gucer et al. 1997; Zargar et al. 2000). A similar approach was tried by Ledger et al., who administered buserelin in a depot preparation for three subsequent months. Elevated gonadotrophin levels, however, rised again after stopping this therapy (Ledger et al. 1989). The same was tried in a prospective placebo-controlled trial by Van Kasteren et al., but it again failed to be successful (van Kasteren et al. 1995). Overall, this approach seems not to be very effective (Buckler et al. 1993), despite anecdotally reported pregnancies (Check et al. 1991).

In a case report, the combination of GnRH agonist administration, ovarian stimulation, and GH supplementation was successful in achieving mature oocytes (Busacca et al. 1996). Using clomifene citrate, ovulations or pregnancies have also been described (Nakai et al. 1984; Davis and Ravnikar 1988). In a prospective trial, danazol was not effective in achieving ovulations in POF pregnancies (Anasti et al. 1994).

In cases of myasthenia gravis, thymectomy with subsequent hormone replacement was successful with regard to achieve a pregnancy in single cases (e.g., Chung et al. 1993).

Since autoimmune disorders can be identified in POF patients, treatment using corticosteroids has been tried and, anecdotally, has been successful. A recent prospective, randomized, placebo-controlled trial, however, did not show any benefit regarding the achievement of ovulation in POF patients (van Kasteren and Schoemaker 1999). This study was planned to include 100 patients, but was closed when in 36 patients no ovulation was found. Patients received in the study arm 9 mg dexamethasone per day and had ovarian stimulation using 300 IU HMG daily. Therefore, corticosteroid treatment seems not to be justified in these patients.

Furthermore, the possible side effects of corticosteroids have to be taken into account, like iatrogenic Cushing's syndrome and osteonecrosis. Both were described in a case report in a patient who got a total dose of 255 mg dexamethasone within a 9-month course of corticosteroids for the treatment of POF (Kalantaridou et al. 1999).

To evaluate the effectiveness of the different described treatment options in POF patients, Van Kasteren and Schoemaker performed a systematic review (van Kasteren and Schoemaker 1999). They could identify a total of 52 case reports, 8 observational studies, 9 uncontrolled studies, and 7 controlled trials. From all the studies, it seems that the chance to conceive for a patient suffering from POF is about 5%–10% after the diagnosis is made.

Interestingly, in the observational studies, 4.8% of patients conceived, in the uncontrolled studies it was 18%, and in the controlled studies 1.5%. Overall the pregnancy rate was 6.3%. This again shows the worth of reliable controlled prospective trials. But since no study showed a significant difference to either placebo or an alternative treatment, is has to be accepted that no treatment can enhance the pregnancy rate.

9.8 Alternative Treatment Options

Besides the treatment options described above, which did not show any benefit at all, three options have to be offered to the patients: adoption, oocyte donation, and surrogate motherhood. The first two are established strategies to help these patients. The latter, however, may only be helpful to a small number of patients, where other options have failed, or no functional uterus is present. There are special ethical considerations which have to be taken into account with this approach, especially the fact of a third involved person, the surrogate mother, as well as the fact that the child will only share half the genetic information with the intending couple – the information of the father. Therefore, it should be up to the physicians and the patients to decide whether this option is suitable or not. In several European countries, surrogate motherhood is forbidden by law.

9.8.1 Oocyte Donation

Oocyte donation describes a therapy in which oocytes from a third persons are retrieved, fertilized by the husbands sperms, and transferred to the patient, who herself does not have functional oocytes available.

Patients who have ovarian infertility due to previous chemo- or radiotherapy apparently have lower success rates from oocyte donation than others (Pados et al. 1992; Franco et al. 1994). This may be also due to damage of the endometrium, which might impair embryo implantation. However, principally the success of oocyte donation in POF patients overall is not different than in patients with another diagnosis – as shown in a retrospective, controlled trial by Lydic et al. (Lydic et al. 1996).

Results of oocyte donation are shown in Table 4 and Fig. 1 (Paulson et al. 1997). Quite promising cumulative pregnancy rates of up to 80%–90% can be reached.

However, oocyte donation has also some ethical problems. There is especially the problem of oocyte source, since only a limited number of women are available to donate oocytes. On the other hand, women, who donate oocytes are paid sometimes more than US $3,000–$5,000. Therefore, some countries, such as the United Kingdom, suggest only

Table 4. Results of oocyte donation according to Marcus and Brinsden 1999

	Cryo-preserved	Patients	Transfer cycles	Clinical pregnancies	Live births
HFEA	No	917	882	259 (29.4%)	201 (22.8%)
HFEA	Yes	298	331	64 (19.3%)	48 (14.5%)
Bourn Hall	Yes	104	107	37 (34.6%)	29 (27.9%)

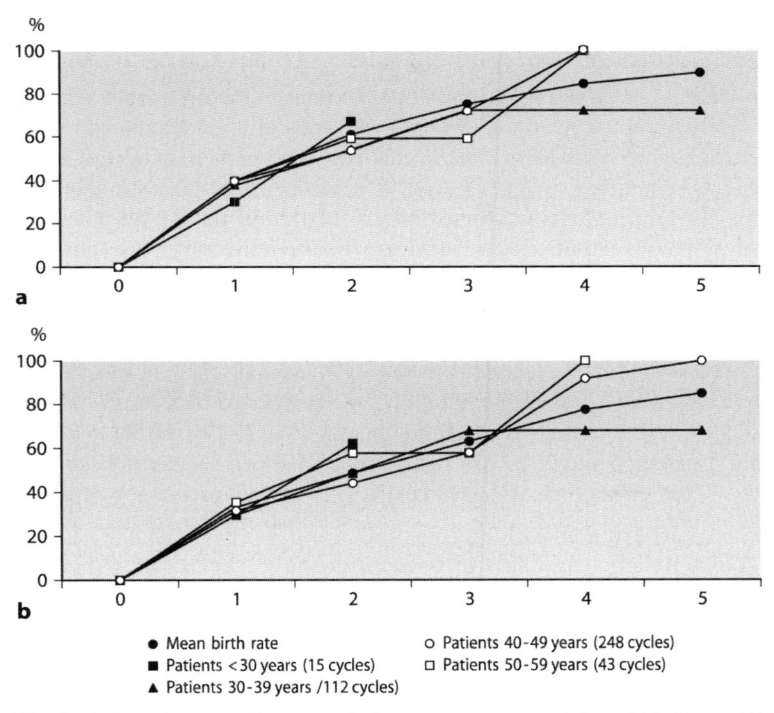

Fig. 1a,b. Results regarding cumulative pregnancy rate (**a**) and birth rate (**b**) after up to five treatment cycles using donated oocytes. Results depending on patients' age are shown. (According to Paulson et al. 1997)

accepting oocyte donation on an altruistic basis. In other countries, like Germany, oocyte donation is forbidden by law (Ludwig and Diedrich 1999, 2000).

To conclude, when oocyte donation is well regulated, it offers a good approach to help patients with ovarian failure to conceive an own child.

9.8.2 Surrogate Motherhood

In the case of surrogate motherhood, a commissioning couple asks for help from a third person – a woman who can carry a pregnancy to term. Surrogate motherhood is done in cases in which a woman herself is not able to become pregnant, e.g., due to removal of the uterus in the past. The ethical problems are more serious than those for oocyte donation. However, in certain cases, surrogate motherhood might be possible without major ethical problems.

Table 5 shows some results regarding the success rates (English et al. 1997). Furthermore, the ASRM report has included results from 64 centers in the U.S.A. These have done 219 cycles in 1994; in 188, oocyte retrieval could be done (85.8%), in 184, an embryo transfer (97.9% of oocyte retrievals). In 61 cases, a pregnancy could be achieved, resulting in a pregnancy rate of 27.8% per cycle, 32.4% per oocyte pick-up, and 33.1% per embryo transfer. However, the multiple pregnancy rate was

Table 5. Results of treatment in assisted reproduction by including surrogate motherhood (according to English et al. 1997)

Couples		27
Stimulation cycles		44
Oocytes retrieved (mean) (range)		9.6 (2–24)
Cryopreserved embryos (mean) (range)		4.7 (1–13)
Surrogate mothers		30
Embryo transfers		40
Transferred embryos (fresh and frozen/thawed) (mean)		2.1
Clinical pregnancies	Per transfer	42.5% (17/40)
	Per surrogate mother	56.7% (17/30)
	Per couple	55.5% (15/27)
Birth rate	Per surrogate mother	41.4% (12/29)
	Per couple	44.4% (12/27)

32.8%, which is a further ethical problem, since it means a severe health problem not only for the children born, but especially under these circumstances for the surrogate mother.

9.8.3 Adoption

The possibility of adoption should be included in each counseling session. Depending on the country, however, this option has a quite low chance of being successful. Especially in Germany, there are much more couples seeking a child for adoption than there are children available.

9.9 Conclusion

Premature ovarian failure means a severe diagnosis for a woman who has not yet finished her family planning. There are different possible causes; most cases, however, remain idiopathic. After diagnosis is made, a spontaneous pregnancy can be achieved in about 5%–10% of cases – as is estimated from controlled, uncontrolled, and observational trials. A treatment option, however, which is able to increase this pregnancy rate, does not exist. The most-used treatment in these cases is oocyte donation. Patients should also be counseled about adoption, and in rare cases, also about surrogate motherhood.

It is very important to focus the interest not only on the problem of premature ovarian failure directly, but also on long-term consequences, like osteoporosis, cardiovascular disease, and other diseases for which these patients are at higher risk. These are, for example, Addison's disease, Diabetes mellitus, and thyroid diseases.

Counseling of siblings of the patients, as well as of other near relatives, is necessary because of a substantial part of genetic causes of this disorder.

References

Aittomaki K, Herva R, Stenman UH, Juntunen K, Ylostalo P, Hovatta O, de la Chapelle A (1996) Clinical features of primary ovarian failure caused by a point mutation in the follicle-stimulating hormone receptor gene. J Clin Endocrinol Metab 81:3722–3726

Allingham-Hawkins DJ, Babul-Hirji R, Chitayat D, Holden JJ, Yang KT, Lee C, Hudson R, Gorwill H, Nolin SL, Glicksman A, Jenkins EC, Brown WT, Howard-Peebles PN, Becchi C, Cummings E, Fallon L, Seitz S, Black SH, Vianna-Morgante AM, Costa SS, Otto PA, Mingroni-Netto RC, Murray A, Webb J, Vieri F (1999) Fragile X premutation is a significant risk factor for premature ovarian failure: the International Collaborative POF in Fragile X study–preliminary data. Am J Med Genet 83:322–325

Alper MM, Garner PR (1985) Premature ovarian failure: its relationship to autoimmune disease. Obstet Gynecol 66:27–30

Amati P, Gasparini P, Zlotogora J, Zelante L, Chomel JC, Kitzis A, Kaplan J, Bonneau D (1996) A gene for premature ovarian failure associated with eyelid malformation maps to chromosome 3q22-q23. Am J Hum Genet 58:1089–1092

Anasti JN (1998) Premature ovarian failure: an update. Fertil Steril 70:1–15

Anasti JN, Kimzey LM, Defensor RA, White B, Nelson LM (1994) A controlled study of danazol for the treatment of karyotypically normal spontaneous premature ovarian failure. Fertil Steril 62:726–730

Anasti JN, Kalantaridou SN, Kimzey LM, Defensor RA, Nelson LM (1998) Bone loss in young women with karyotypically normal spontaneous premature ovarian failure. Obstet Gynecol 91:12–15

Arif S, Vallian S, Farzaneh F, Zanone MM, James SL, Pietropaolo M, Hettiarachchi S, Vergani D, Conway GS, Peakman M (1996) Identification of 3 beta-hydroxysteroid dehydrogenase as a novel target of steroid cell autoantibodies: association of autoantibodies with endocrine autoimmune disease. J Clin Endocrinol Metab 81:4439–4445

Beau I, Touraine P, Meduri G, Gougeon A, Desroches A, Matuchansky C, Milgrom E, Kuttenn F, Misrahi M (1998) A novel phenotype related to partial loss of function mutations of the follicle stimulating hormone receptor. J Clin Invest 102:1352–1359

Belvisi L, Bombelli F, Sironi L, Doldi N (1993) Organ-specific autoimmunity in patients with premature ovarian failure. J Endocrinol Invest 16:889–892

Betterle C, Rossi A, Dalla PS, Artifoni A, Pedini B, Gavasso S, Caretto A (1993) Premature ovarian failure: autoimmunity and natural history. Clin Endocrinol (Oxf) 39:35–43

Blumenfeld Z, Avivi I (1999) Trying to preserve ovarian function in the face of chemotherapy? [letter; comment]. Fertil Steril 71:773–775

Blumenfeld Z, Avivi I, Linn S, Epelbaum R, Ben-Shahar M, Haim N (1996) Prevention of irreversible chemotherapy-induced ovarian damage in young women with lymphoma by a gonadotrophin-releasing hormone agonist in parallel to chemotherapy. Hum Reprod 11:1620–1626

Blumenfeld Z, Haim N (1997) Prevention of gonadal damage during cytotoxic therapy. Ann Med 29:199–206

Buckler HM, Healy DL, Burger HG (1993) Does gonadotropin suppression result in follicular development in premature ovarian failure? Gynecol Endocrinol 7:123–128

Busacca M, Fusi FM, Brigante C, Doldi N, Vignali M (1996) Success in inducing ovulation in a case of premature ovarian failure using growth hormone-releasing hormone. Gynecol Endocrinol 10:277–279

Check JH, Chase JS, Spence M (1989) Pregnancy in premature ovarian failure after therapy with oral contraceptives despite resistance to previous human menopausal gonadotropin therapy. Am J Obstet Gynecol 160:114–115

Check JH, Nowroozi K, Nazari A (1991) Viable pregnancy in a woman with premature ovarian failure treated with gonadotropin suppression and human menopausal gonadotropin stimulation. A case report. J Reprod Med 36:195–197

Chen FP, Chang SY (1997) Spontaneous pregnancy in patients with premature ovarian failure. Acta Obstet Gynecol Scand 76:81–82

Chung TK, Haines CJ, Yip SK (1993) Case report: spontaneous pregnancy following thymectomy for myasthenia gravis associated with premature ovarian failure. Asia Oceania J Obstet Gynaecol 19:253–255

Conway GS, Hettiarachchi S, Murray A, Jacobs PA (1995) Fragile X premutations in familial premature ovarian failure. Lancet 346:309–310

Conway GS, Kaltsas G, Patel A, Davies MC, Jacobs HS (1996) Characterization of idiopathic premature ovarian failure. Fertil Steril 65:337–341

Conway GS, Payne NN, Webb J, Murray A, Jacobs PA (1998) Fragile X premutation screening in women with premature ovarian failure. Hum Reprod 13:1184–1187

Coulam CB, Adamson SC, Annegers JF (1986) Incidence of premature ovarian failure. Obstet Gynecol 67:604–606

Davis OK, Ravnikar VA (1988) Ovulation induction with clomiphene citrate in a women with premature ovarian failure. A case report. J Reprod Med 33:559–562

Davison RM, Quilter CR, Webb J, Murray A, Fisher AM, Valentine A, Serhal P, Conway GS (1998) A familial case of X chromosome deletion ascertained by cytogenetic screening of women with premature ovarian failure. Hum Reprod 13:3039–3041

de Moraes RM, Blizzard RM, Garcia-Bunuel R, Jones GS (1972) Autoimmunity and ovarian failure. Am J Obstet Gynecol 112:693–703

Devi AS, Metzger DA, Luciano AA, Benn PA (1998) 45,X/46,XX mosaicism in patients with idiopathic premature ovarian failure. Fertil Steril 70:89–93

English V, Sommerville A, Brinsden P (1997) Surrogacy. In: Shenfield F, Sureau C (eds) Ethical dilemmas in assisted reproduction. Parthenon Publishing Group, New York, pp 31–40

Fenichel P, Sosset C, Barbarino-Monnier P, Gobert B, Hieronimus S, Bene MC, Harter M (1997) Prevalence, specificity and significance of ovarian antibodies during spontaneous premature ovarian failure. Hum Reprod 12:2623–2628

Fonte Kohek MB, Batista MC, Russell AJ, Vass K, Giacaglia LR, Mendonca BB, Latronico AC (1998) No evidence of the inactivating mutation (C566T) in the follicle-stimulating hormone receptor gene in Brazilian women with premature ovarian failure. Fertil Steril 70:565–567

Franco JG Jr, Baruffi RL, Mauri AL, Pertersen CG, Campos MS, Oliveira JB (1994) Donation of oocytes as treatment for infertility in patients with premature ovarian failure. Awarded the "Nicolau de Moraes Barros" prize for gynecology. Rev Paul Med 112:510–516

Gobert B, Barabarino-Monnier P, Guillet-Rosso F, Bene MC, Faure GC (1990) Ovary antibodies after IVF. Lancet 335:723

Golonka JE, Goodman AD (1968) Coexistence of primary ovarian insufficiency, primary adrenocortical insufficiency and idiopathic hypoparathyroidism. J Clin Endocrinol Metab 28:79–82

Gucer F, Urdl W, Pieber D, Arikan MG, Giuliani A, Auner H (1997) Pregnancies in patients with premature ovarian failure. Clin Exp Obstet Gynecol 24:130–132

Guerrero NV, Singh RH, Manatunga A, Berry GT, Steiner RD, Elsas LJ (2000) Risk factors for premature ovarian failure in females with galactosemia. J Pediatr 137:833–841

Hundscheid RD, Sistermans EA, Thomas CM, Braat DD, Straatman H, Kiemeney LA, Oostra BA, Smits AP (2000) Imprinting effect in premature ovarian failure confined to paternally inherited fragile X premutations. Am J Hum Genet 66:413–418

Irvine WJ, Chan MM, Scarth L, Kolb FO, Hartog M, Bayliss RI, Drury MI (1968) Immunological aspects of premature ovarian failure associated with idiopathic Addison's disease. Lancet 2:883–887

Kalantaridou SN, Braddock DT, Patronas NJ, Nelson LM (1999) Treatment of autoimmune premature ovarian failure. Hum Reprod 14:1777–1782

Kim TJ, Anasti JN, Flack MR, Kimzey LM, Defensor RA, Nelson LM (1997) Routine endocrine screening for patients with karyotypically normal spontaneous premature ovarian failure. Obstet Gynecol 89:777–779

Krauss CM, Turksoy RN, Atkins L, McLaughlin C, Brown LG, Page DC (1987) Familial premature ovarian failure due to an interstitial deletion of the long arm of the X chromosome. N Engl J Med 317:125–131

Kuki S, Morgan RL, Tucci JR (1981) Myasthenia gravis and premature ovarian failure. Arch Intern Med 141:1230–1232

Ledger WL, Thomas EJ, Browning D, Lenton EA, Cooke ID (1989) Suppression of gonadotrophin secretion does not reverse premature ovarian failure. Br J Obstet Gynaecol 96:196–199

Leeton J, Rogers P, Cameron I, Caro C, Healy D (1989) Pregnancy results following embryo transfer in women receiving low-dosage variable-length estrogen replacement therapy for premature ovarian failure. J In Vitro Fert Embryo Transf 6:232–235

Letterie G, Miyazawa K (1989) A combination of gonadotropin-releasing hormone analog and human menopausal gonadotropins for ovulation induction in premature ovarian failure. Acta Obstet Gynecol Scand 68:571–573

Luborsky JL, Visintin I, Boyers S, Asari T, Caldwell B, DeCherney A (1990) Ovarian antibodies detected by immobilized antigen immunoassay in patients with premature ovarian failure. J Clin Endocrinol Metab 70:69–75

Ludwig M, Diedrich K (1999) Regulation of assisted reproductive technology: the German experience. In: Brinsden PR (ed) A textbook of in vitro fertilization and assisted reproduction. Parthenon Publishing Group, New York, pp 431–434

Ludwig M, Diedrich K (2000) Ethical problems of the German embryo protection law. Ref Gynecol Obstet 7:1–6

Lutjen PJ, Findlay JK, Trounson AO, Leeton JF, Chan LK (1986) Effect on plasma gonadotropins of cyclic steroid replacement in women with premature ovarian failure. J Clin Endocrinol Metab 62:419–423

Lydic ML, Liu JH, Rebar RW, Thomas MA, Cedars MI (1996) Success of donor oocyte in in vitro fertilization-embryo transfer in recipients with and without premature ovarian failure. Fertil Steril 65:98–102

Marcus SF, Brinsden PR (1999) Oocyte donation. In: Brinsden PR (ed) A textbook of in vitro fertilization and assisted reproduction. Parthenon Publishing Group, New York, pp 343-345

Marozzi A, Vegetti W, Manfredini E, Tibiletti MG, Testa G, Crosignani PG, Ginelli E, Meneveri R, Dalpra L (2000) Association between idiopathic premature ovarian failure and fragile X premutation. Hum Reprod 15:197–202

Menashe Y, Pearlstone AC, Surrey ES (1996) Spontaneous pregnancies despite failed attempts at ovulation induction in a woman with latrogenic premature ovarian failure. J Reprod Med 41:207–210

Murray A, Ennis S, Morton N (2000) No evidence for parent of origin influencing premature ovarian failure in fragile X premutation carriers. Am J Hum Genet 67:253–254

Nakai M, Tatsumi H, Arai M (1984) Case report. Successive pregnancies in a patient with premature ovarian failure. Eur J Obstet Gynecol Reprod Biol 18:217–224

Ohsawa M, Wu MC, Masahashi T, Asai M, Narita O (1985) Cyclic therapy resulted in pregnancy in premature ovarian failure. Obstet Gynecol 66:64S–67S

Olivar AC (1996) The role of laparoscopic ovarian biopsy in the management of premature gonadal failure. Conn Med 60:707–708

Pados G, Camus M, Van Waesberghe L, Liebaers I, Van Steirteghem A, Devroey P (1992) Oocyte and embryo donation: evaluation of 412 consecutive trials. Hum Reprod 7:1111–1117

Paulson RJ, Hatch IE, Lobo RA, Sauer MV (1997) Cumulative conception and live birth rates after oocyte donation: implications regarding endometrial receptivity. Hum Reprod 12:835–839

Powell CM, Taggart RT, Drumheller TC, Wangsa D, Qian C, Nelson LM, White BJ (1994) Molecular and cytogenetic studies of an X; autosome translocation in a patient with premature ovarian failure and review of the literature. Am J Med Genet 52:19–26

Sala C, Arrigo G, Torri G, Martinazzi F, Riva P, Larizza L, Philippe C, Jonveaux P, Sloan F, Labella T, Toniolo D (1997) Eleven X chromosome breakpoints associated with premature ovarian failure (POF) map to a 15-Mb YAC contig spanning Xq21. Genomics 40:123–131

Shelling AN, Burton KA, Chand AL, van Ee CC, France JT, Farquhar CM, Milsom SR, Love DR, Gersak K, Aittomaki K, Winship IM (2000) Inhibin: a candidate gene for premature ovarian failure. Hum Reprod 15:2644–2649

Sherman SL (2000) Premature ovarian failure among fragile X premutation carriers: parent-of-origin effect? Am J Hum Genet 67:11–13

Sheu BC, Ho HN, Yang YS (1996) Spontaneous pregnancy after previous pregnancy by oocyte donation due to premature ovarian failure. Hum Reprod 11:1359–1360

Smith HC, Seale JP, Posen S (1974) Premature ovarian failure in a triple X female. J Obstet Gynaecol Br Commonw 81:405–409

Snick HK, Snick TS, Evers JL, Collins JA (1997) The spontaneous pregnancy prognosis in untreated subfertile couples: the Walcheren primary care study. Hum Reprod 12:1582–1588

Sung L, Bustillo M, Mukherjee T, Booth G, Karstaedt A, Copperman AB (1997) Sisters of women with premature ovarian failure may not be ideal ovum donors. Fertil Steril 67:912–916

Takakura K, Takebayashi K, Wang HQ, Kimura F, Kasahara K, Noda Y (2001) Follicle-stimulating hormone receptor gene mutations are rare in Japanese women with premature ovarian failure and polycystic ovary syndrome. Fertil Steril 75:207–209

Takebayashi K, Takakura K, Wang H, Kimura F, Kasahara K, Noda Y (2000) Mutation analysis of the growth differentiation factor-9 and –9B genes in patients with premature ovarian failure and polycystic ovary syndrome. Fertil Steril 74:976–979

Tang L, Sawers RS (1989) Twin pregnancy in premature ovarian failure after estrogen treatment: a case report. Am J Obstet Gynecol 161:172–173

Tharapel AT, Anderson KP, Simpson JL, Martens PR, Wilroy RS Jr, Llerena JC Jr, Schwartz CE (1993) Deletion (X) (q26.1–q28) in a proband and her mother: molecular characterization and phenotypic-karyotypic deductions. Am J Hum Genet 52:463–471

Tong Y, Liao WX, Roy AC, Ng SC (2001) Absence of mutations in the coding regions of follicle-stimulating hormone receptor gene in Singapore Chinese women with premature ovarian failure and polycystic ovary syndrome. Horm Metab Res 33:221–226

Touraine P, Beau I, Gougeon A, Meduri G, Desroches A, Pichard C, Detoeuf M, Paniel B, Prieur M, Zorn JR, Milgrom E, Kuttenn F, Misrahi M (1999) New natural inactivating mutations of the follicle-stimulating hormone receptor: correlations between receptor function and phenotype. Mol Endocrinol 13:1844–1854

Turkington RW, Lebovitz HE (1967) Extra-adrenal endocrine deficiencies in Addison's disease. Am J Med 43:499–507

Uzielli ML, Guarducci S, Lapi E, Cecconi A, Ricci U, Ricotti G, Biondi C, Scarselli B, Vieri F, Scarnato P, Gori F, Sereni A (1999) Premature ovarian failure (POF) and fragile X premutation females: from POF to fragile X carrier identification, from fragile X carrier diagnosis to POF association data. Am J Med Genet 84:300–303

van Kasteren YM, Schoemaker J (1999) Premature ovarian failure: a systematic review on therapeutic interventions to restore ovarian function and achieve pregnancy. Hum Reprod Update 5:483–492

van Kasteren YM, Hoek A, Schoemaker J (1995) Ovulation induction in premature ovarian failure: a placebo-controlled randomized trial combining pituitary suppression with gonadotropin stimulation. Fertil Steril 64:273–278

van Kasteren YM, Braat DD, Hemrika DJ, Lambalk CB, Rekers-Mombarg LT, von Blomberg BM, Schoemaker J (1999a) Corticosteroids do not influence ovarian responsiveness to gonadotropins in patients with premature ovarian failure: a randomized, placebo-controlled trial. Fertil Steril 71:90–95

van Kasteren YM, Hundscheid RD, Smits AP, Cremers FP, van Zonneveld P, Braat DD (1999b) Familial idiopathic premature ovarian failure: an overrated and underestimated genetic disease? Hum Reprod 14:2455–2459

Vazquez AM, Kenny FM (1973) Ovarian failure and antiovarian antibodies in association with hypoparathyroidism, moniliasis, and Addison's and Hashimoto's diseases. Obstet Gynecol 41:414–418

Vegetti W, Grazia TM, Testa G, de Lauretis Y, Alagna F, Castoldi E, Taborelli M, Motta T, Bolis PF, Dalpra L, Crosignani PG (1998) Inheritance in idiopathic premature ovarian failure: analysis of 71 cases. Hum Reprod 13:1796–1800

Vianna-Morgante AM, Costa SS (2000) Premature ovarian failure is associated with maternally and paternally inherited premutation in Brazilian families with fragile X. Am J Hum Genet 67:254–255

Villanueva AL, Rebar RW (1983) Triple-X syndrome and premature ovarian failure. Obstet Gynecol 62:70s–73s

Whitney EA, Layman LC, Chan PJ, Lee A, Peak DB, McDonough PG (1995) The follicle-stimulating hormone receptor gene is polymorphic in premature ovarian failure and normal controls. Fertil Steril 64:518–524

Williams RS, Littell RD, Mendenhall NP (1999) Laparoscopic oophoropexy and ovarian function in the treatment of Hodgkin disease. Cancer 86:2138–2142

Zargar AH, Salahuddin M, Wani AI, Bashir MI, Masoodi SR, Laway BA (2000) Pregnancy in premature ovarian failure: a possible role of estrogen plus progesterone treatment. J Assoc Physicians India 48:213–215

10 Can Stimulation Protocols Improve Oocyte Quality?

J. Smitz

10.1 Introduction 161
10.2 The Development of Human In Vitro Maturation of Oocytes 163
10.3 Patient Selection for In Vitro Maturation 164
10.4 The Health Record of Small Antral (Immature) Follicles 165
10.5 Kinetics of FSH and Follicle Development 167
10.6 Strategies of Patient Pretreatment Before Immature Oocyte Pick-up 168
10.7 Conclusions 171
References 171

10.1 Introduction

Ovarian follicle development in humans is a lengthy process that takes several months. Initial follicle recruitment from the resting pool is regulated by intraovarian factors and independent of circulating gonadotropin concentrations. Once follicles have initiated growth, they progress through a slow preantral growth phase (approximately 4 months) during which the formation of zona pellucida, granulosa cell layers, theca cell layers, and vascularization of the theca externa are accomplished (for review, see Richards 2001). The preantral growth stages are mainly under paracrine/autocrine control but the somatic cells already express the receptors for gonadotropins (Sokka et al. 1996; Oktay et al. 1997). Although the growth of preantral follicles are considered to be gonadotropin-independent, there are arguments that gonadotropin fluctuations may effect these early growing follicles (Parrot and Skinner 1998a,b). Along the lengthy track of follicle growth, granulosa cells are stimulated by a variety of factors such as epidermal growth factor (EGF), insulin-like growth factor-1 (IGF-1), basic fibroblast growth factor (bFGF), transforming growth factor α (TGF-α) and keratinocyte growth factor (KGF).

FSH and LH become essential survival factors for follicles that start to form an antral cavity. Tonic gonadotropin levels are required to enable follicles to reach 2–5 mm diameter and to develop an antrum. During the cyclic increases of follicle-stimulating hormone (FSH), the cohort of antral follicles of 2–5 mm diameter is stimulated for further growth (Gougeon 1996). Absence of FSH at this moment of follicular development leads to spontaneous follicular apoptosis. It is the intercycle FSH rise which will progressively induce both aromatase and LH receptor expression within granulosa cells of the growing units. Further growth of the cohort beyond the early follicular phase up to the preovulatory phase (during the first half of the menstrual cycle) will become supported by several overlapping regulatory pathways leading to follicular dominance. It has been demonstrated that the natural mechanism of follicular dominance results from the increased sensitivity of the leading follicle to the decreasing FSH serum concentrations resulting from the feedback action of estradiol (E_2) secreted by the largest follicle (Zeleznik and Kubik 1986). The increased sensitivity is driven by a series of paracrine events involving androgens, IGF-I, activin/inhibin and their binding proteins (for review see Armstrong and Webb 1997; Hillier and Tetsuka 1997; Ethier and Findlay 2001).

Folliculogenesis in the human ovary is a very inefficient process: far less than 1% of all follicles initiating growth will finally become preovulatory and able to shed a fully grown fertilizable oocyte. The mechanisms by which this follicle reaches its endpoint can be described as "being at the right time at the right place" or by the ability of the somatic cells to survive upon receipt of apoptotic signals. Within the follicle cells cell death inducers (p53, FAS, Fas Ligand, caspases) and survival factors (Bcl-2, inhibitor of apoptosis protein) are constitutively present. These factors can be mobilized and their relative balance determines the fate of the follicle (Asselin et al. 2000).

Ovulation induction and superovulation within assisted reproduction treatment have rapidly evolved in the last decades. The development of pure gonadotropin preparations and of analogs of gonadotropin-releasing hormone (GnRH) have aided clinical research in understanding how antral follicle growth is regulated by FSH and LH during the 14 days before ovulation. In vitro fertilization (IVF) of a series of mature oocytes and the replacement of two to three embryos can considerably increase the chances of conception in infertile women. Superovulation has, however, some serious drawbacks such as the life-threatening ovarian hyperstimulation syndrome and the prolonged use of high doses of reproductive hormones [FSH, LH, human chorionic gonadotropin (HCG)] and related drugs (GnRH agonists, GnRH antagonists, progesterone, estrogens) makes infertility treatment notoriously burdensome for women (Rizk and Smitz 1992).

In an attempt to avoid serious complications and to make IVF more "women-friendly" alternative protocols have been pioneered aiming for drug reduction and shorter treatment duration (Hildebrandt et al. 2001).

10.2 The Development of Human In Vitro Maturation of Oocytes

A potentially valid alternative could be "in vitro maturation" (IVM) (Trounson et al. 1994). Instead of aspirating oocyte–cumulus complexes (OCC) out of preovulatory large follicles (15–22 mm diameter) obtained after a variable stimulation period, the goal is to retrieve OCC out of small (6–12 mm diameter) follicles after a minimal drug therapeutic intervention (for review see Smitz et al. 2001). In order to obtain acceptable results in terms of pregnancies per treatment cycle, this new approach has to be optimized on all fronts: patient selection criteria, ovarian stimulation pretreatment regime, the aspiration technology, the oocyte in vitro maturation technique, the assisted fertilization and embryo culture methods and last but not least the endometrial preparation before embryo transfer. As published today, clinical results state that embryo implantation rates from IVM treatments are only one third of those from conventional IVF treatments (Chian et al. 2000). The current chapter discusses how one could improve the number as well as the quality of the oocytes aspirated from small follicles and questions whether ovarian stimulation treatment could be helpful in achieving this.

10.3 Patient Selection for In Vitro Maturation

Considering the fact that culture techniques of immature OCC are (as yet) not providing equivalent quality embryos as mature OCC, it is very important at present to perform a selection of women who could benefit from this novel treatment.

The best predictions of ovarian follicle recruitment by gonadotropins for IVF in normo-ovulatory women are transvaginal ultrasound on the fifth day after start of menses in the cycle immediately preceding IVF and serum androstenedione concentration on day 6 (Dumesic et al. 2001). Other early biomarkers of poor ovarian response are serum basal FSH on day 3 (Scott et al. 1989), high serum FSH/LH ratio on day 3 (Barroso et al. 2001), and combinations of FSH, inhibin B and estradiol (Seifer et al. 1999).

Analysis of IVM reports leads to conclusions on predictors for success (that are also true for normal IVF patients): the more oocytes that can be retrieved from a patient, the higher are the chances for conception in that treatment cycle. The largest amounts of OCC can be obtained from polycystic ovarian disease (PCOD)-like patients and the best results in terms of clinical pregnancy are observed in this group. The PCO population is also attractive for this kind of study on the sole theoretical basis that in PCOD normal progression of follicle growth beyond 10–12 mm is compromised. Isolation of these OCC and further maturation outside a cystic follicle has a rationale to save the oocyte cumulus from atresia within the cystic follicle.

Results of IVM from oocyte collection in normal women or poor responders do very often not lead to a harvest of over five oocyte cumulus complexes. This modest recovery obviously compromises the chances to have enough good-quality embryos for transfer. A recent publication from Mikkelsen and Lindenberg (2001) reported a series of 100 consecutive IVM treatment cycles performed in PCO (n=29) and normo-ovulatory women (n=71). The PCO patients were stimulated with 150 IU/day for 3 days with Gonal-F (Serono) initiated on day 3 and were aspirated on day 8–9. The group of normo-ovulatory women was unstimulated. A total number of 481 cumulus-enclosed oocytes were obtained in the 100 cycles of which a mean of 55% completed meiosis. The mean number of MII oocytes obtained after IVM from the PCO group was 3.24 and for the normo-ovulatory women 2.4. There was no difference in morphological grading between the two patient populations, and 50% of all oocytes appeared to have no anomalies. These results show that although the recovery rates are lower in normo-ovulatory women compared to PCO in a group of selected patients (younger than 37 years and only good responders testified by eventual previous IVF treatment), maturation, fertilization, preimplantation oocyte development, and pregnancy rate per cycle were not different between both groups. On average, 60% of these oocytes fertilized normally, 50% cleaved and from 12% of the cycles ensued a pregnancy. This study related oocyte morphology to embryo quality after in vitro maturation and fertilization and reported no higher frequency of oocyte anomalies in IVM oocytes than after conventional IVF or ICSI stimulation.

10.4 The Health Record of Small Antral (Immature) Follicles

Theoretically, one could plan oocyte retrieval from small (6–12 mm) follicles at any moment of the menstrual life. However, as gonadotropins experience cyclic changes during the cycle, these fluctuations are expected to have a firm impact on follicle health. Studies from McNatty et al. (1979), who studied surgically removed whole human ovaries from women aged 25–49 years, indicated that the average number of antral follicles (≥4 mm diameter) from both ovaries was 14 or less. Somewhat more than 10% of the follicles of this study contained the full complement of granulosa cells, predicting an availability of only 1 to 2 oocytes for further culture and IVF. McNatty stated that at the onset of the follicular phase of the menstrual cycle, the largest non-atretic follicle had reached a diameter of 4 mm and that selection of the ovulatory follicle is likely to be made some time before the onset of the follicular phase. From the data on human ovarian tissue from Gougeon (1986), it is known that atretic changes can be found in all follicle classes, but that classes of 5 and 6, in particular, show a high proportion of atretic follicles. A study from Yuan and Giudice (1997) analyzed the frequency of follicular apoptosis in ovaries from normal cycling women and found the highest frequency in the class of small antral follicles with a diameter between 2 and 10 mm. A recent publication of Mikkelsen et al. (2001) reports on the occurrence of apoptosis in follicular aspirates from small antral follicles from unstimulated normal women and from superovulated normal and PCO women. Apoptosis as measured by the APOPTAG kit (Intergen, Oxford, UK) revealed a median rate of apoptosis of 46% in unstimulated normal women. Ovarian stimulation during 3 days with recombinant (r)FSH (150 IU/day), starting 3 days after onset of menses reduced this rate of apoptosis by half. It was noteworthy that PCO women had a rate of apoptosis of 41%, despite their exposure to rFSH treatment. In this paper, Mikkelsen also describes whether occurrence of follicular dominance (in one ovary) has an impact on the apoptosis rate in the companion follicles of the ipsilateral ovary compared to the contralateral ovary. Surprisingly, presence of a leading follicle did not cause inhibition (by paracrine mechanisms) on the companion follicles: instead, apoptosis remained lower than in the contralateral ovary (42% vs 59% respectively). Although in the study of Mikkelsen, apoptosis did differ in accordance to stimulation or presence of a dominant follicle; this had apparently no significant impact on the quality of the oocyte and its further developmental competence after fertilization. It can be concluded that the target group of follicles for IVM in humans is sensitive to apoptotic changes. This is not particular for the human species as, similar to domestic species, 85% of antral follicles in an ovary at any time of the cycle show signs of atresia (Driancourt 1991; Pavlok et al. 1992). Results from human IVF have claimed that oocytes had a better developmental competence when apoptosis in cumulus and mural granulosa was only present at a low incidence (Nakahara et al. 1997; Host et al. 2000). This finding is in contradiction with reports in cattle from Blondin and Sirard (1995), who stressed even better developmental competence by retrieving OCC out of follicles with signs of onset of atresia.

Pretreatment with gonadotropins in view of an IVM treatment has not shown unequivocally beneficial results (Mikkelsen et al. 1999). In animal species, gonadotropin pretreatment enhanced meiotic maturation in vitro in cat, pig, sheep, and bovine (Johnston et al. 1989; Younis et al. 1989; Galli and Moor 1991; Mattioli et al. 1991). In bovine, Lu et al. (1991) reported a higher inner cell mass in blastocysts after IVM of oocytes retrieved from FSH-primed animals compared to untreated ones. In rhesus monkeys, Schramm and Bavister (1994) reported positive effects of FSH priming on oocyte competence. More recent experiments from Sirard et al. (1999) in cattle emphasized that the dose of

FSH (decreasing doses) and the timing of follicle aspiration (time interval between last FSH dose and follicle aspiration) are critical factors determining oocyte developmental competence. These data reiterated their previous findings that a subtle degree of atresia in small follicles (induced by FSH deprivation) could initiate stimuli important for further developmental competence. In a pilot study by Mikkelsen et al. (1998), there was also an improved oocyte maturation rate after FSH priming when follicle aspiration was delayed up to 72 h instead of 24 h after the last FSH dose.

10.5 Kinetics of FSH and Follicle Development

There is a good rationale to find therapeutic techniques to prevent the occurrence of atresia in this follicle class by using potent inducers of growth such as gonadotropins.

A number of small antral follicles candidate for assisted reproduction techniques (ART) are present well before the onset of the follicular phase of the treatment cycle and their survival is mainly dependent on rising FSH levels during the luteo-follicular transition. Brown (1978) suggested that an elevation of FSH concentrations of 10%–30% above threshold level stimulated normal mono-ovulation, while a further increase provoked multiple follicle development. Baird (1987) has in addition proposed the "FSH-gate" concept adding the notion of time during which FSH concentrations stay above threshold levels. It was demonstrated recently in humans by Schipper et al. (1998) that already gentle interference with the decrease of FSH provokes multiple follicle development. The study by Schipper et al. (1998) demonstrated that a single high (375 IU rFSH) dose of FSH to regularly cycling women at the onset of menses induced increased growth of small antral follicles during subsequent days, but did not affect dominant follicle growth beyond 10-mm follicles. It has been well documented by Lass et al. (1997) that the number and quality of antral follicles present during the luteo-follicular transition is dependent on the age of the patient (total follicular content). Less well clear are the influences of eventually previous medical interventions such as pituitary desensitization pretreatment, luteal phase supplementation, multiple ovulation in the preceding cycle, and eventual hormonal contraceptive use.

10.6 Strategies of Patient Pretreatment Before Immature Oocyte Pick-up

The target follicles to aspirate for IVM have a follicle diameter between 6 and 12 mm. Previous studies have demonstrated that follicles smaller than 6 mm are less often meiotically competent and this follicle diameter corresponds to the lower limit of follicle diameter of which the oocyte did give rise to blastocyst formation (Trounson et al. 2001). From follicles larger than 12 mm diameter, often no OCC can be aspirated (Albano et al. 2001). Furthermore, it is aimed to ideally retrieve OCC from a well-synchronized cohort of follicle diameters. Progression of growth of the gonadotropin-dependent stages is dependent on the variability of FSH intercycle increase, which is modulated by the CL regression or eventual previous cycle treatment regimen. Follicular homogeneity is very much dependent on the follicular reserve (patient's age) and on timely and sustained increases of intercyclic FSH. In view of IVM, one should only decide to go for oocyte pick-up if there is sign of a well-synchronized cohort of follicles and plan the day of retrieval when the largest follicles reach a mean follicle diameter of 12 mm. Experience from conventional superovulation using GnRH agonists in desensitization protocols followed by gonadotropin stimulation emphasizes the advantages of working with cycle programming. Management of superovulation in view of ART gained many benefits by abolishment of patients' own gonadotropin secretion, as well at the start of the cycle (FSH low) as on the days preceding ovulation (LH low). Large IVF/ICSI registries illustrated superior results by applying GnRH analogs in desensitization (long) protocols (for review see Schats and Schoemaker 2001). The improved results in comparison to other [no GnRH agonists, GnRH antagonists, short (flare-up) GnRH agonist] stimulation regimens could be due to beneficial effects at different levels of the treatment procedure such as (1) the nature of selection of the follicle cohort, (2) the continuous endogenous LH depletion before ovulation, and/or (3) an improved endometrial environment for implantation or a combination of previous factors. The degree of variability of the intercycle FSH rises can be reduced by creating a hypogonadotropic state using either GnRH analogs or steroids (contraceptives). Both possibilities have been explored with success; however, the use of a contraceptive oestro-progestative pill is undoubtedly more comfortable and less costly for the patient (de Ziegler et al. 1998). After a period of hypogonadotropism, follicles that became FSH dependent can be hit subsequently with a sufficiently high FSH dose to surpass the threshold and to remain bioavailable for a number of days. The FSH stimulus should be potent enough to override other intraovarian paracrine/autocrine regulatory mechanisms potentially involved in atresia. Although many of the aforementioned strategies have been used, there are as yet insufficient data available from prospective studies allowing to propose a first-choice regimen to optimize oocyte recovery. Regarding the type of gonadotropin, mixture studies are also missing. It is as yet unclear whether there is a need to have supplements of LH at start of stimulation or whether this supplementation should be restricted mainly to severely gonadotropin-depleted conditions. In view of the build-up of a receptive endometrium, there should be a sufficiently long E_2 impregnation phase. Availability of LH might be crucial to ensure thecal androgen production, which is at the basis of the transformation of estrogen production.

Recent studies by our group (unpublished observations) illustrate the relation between sufficiently recovered gonadotropin levels after suppression by contraceptive pill use and the build-up of a critical amount of circulatory E_2 for endometrial maturation.

As shown by Schipper et al. (1998), a single high FSH dose administered at onset of menses in normal cycling women provoked only a modest and unsustained increase of E_2 concentrations, making E_2 supplementation almost surely a must for endometrial build-up. At present, usefulness of ovarian stimulation for immature follicle aspiration is still controversial. The studies reporting IVM practice have, to date, not convincingly shown whether gonadotropins can really improve oocyte developmental competence.

Although data from animal experiments are rather favoring the use of FSH pretreatment, there are as yet not enough data to claim that this is also true for humans. Indeed, as illustrated in Table 1, fair numbers of COC can be retrieved from unstimulated ovaries, especially in PCO like patients. In normal cycling women, the study of Mikkelsen et al. (2001) did not report significant improvement by using FSH. However, in PCO patients, Mikkelsen and Lindenberg (2001) found a clear improvement on the maturational potential and implantation rate by using recombinant FSH pretreatment. It is worthwhile to comment on the interesting

Table 1. Number of oocyte cumuli obtained after aspiration of small immature follicles. Results are shown for polycystic ovarian disease (PCOD), normo-ovulatory women and in relation to FSH stimulation

Author	Patients	Cycle	Number oocytes aspirated
Cha et al. 1991	Normal	Natural	12
Cha and Chian 1998	PCOD	Natural	12.6
Trounson et al. 1994	PCOD	Natural	12–15
	Normal	Natural	2.8
Barnes 1996	PCOD	Natural	16.5
	Normal	Natural	4.9
Russell et al. 1997	Mixed	Natural	11.5
Wynn et al. 1998	Normal	Natural	3.7
	Normal	Stimulated	7.7
Mikkelsen 1999 et al.	Normal	Natural	3.7
	Normal	Stimulated	3.7
Cobo et al. 1999	Normal	Natural	4.9–6.8
Smith et al. 2000	Normal	Natural	5–6
Mikkelsen et al. 2001a	Normal	Unstimulated	4
	Normal	Stimulated	7
Mikkelsen et al. 2001b	PCOD	Stimulated	6
	Normal	Unstimulated	4
Child et al. 2001	PCOD	Unstimulated	10.3

findings from Chian et al. (2000). These authors found a clear benefit in terms of clinical pregnancy results by retrieving OCC out of small immature follicles after injecting HCG. Apparently, this trigger before aspiration of small follicles initiates a biochemical program, which favors further oocyte development after in vitro maturation. As we would not expect such a small follicle (<12 mm diameter) to express the LH receptor on the mural granulosa at this stage, one could speculate that HCG might be influencing the theca compartment which could effect granulosa cell and oocyte maturation in a paracrine way (Parrott and Skinner 1998a,b). Child et al. (2001) reported an implantation rate of 9.5% by immature oocyte retrieval from unstimulated cycles in PCO patients by applying a HCG injection before oocyte aspiration.

10.7 Conclusions

Gonadotropins are major drivers of the ovarian follicle. Full developmental competence of the oocyte is acquired during the last stages of the antral growth phase, which is driven by the delicate balance of FSH and LH. Through the somatic compartment consisting of theca and differentiated granulosa cells which are expressing receptors for LH and FSH in a sequential manner, both gonadotropins can exert influences on the oocyte. The relative importance of the different components in human ovarian folliculogenesis has been clarified by using GnRH agonists in combination with different proportions of recombinant gonadotropins. This knowledge can now be used to adapt current stimulation practice in the way that assisted reproduction treatment becomes more safe and women friendly. The development of IVM still needs optimization from the side of patient pretreatment by gonadotropins. More research is needed to optimize in vitro maturation culture conditions. Oocyte viability in vitro is dependent on a complex interaction of biochemical signals that need to be delivered to an oocyte–cumulus unit in a correct sequential timing and concentration.

References

Albano C, Platteau P, Nogueira D, Cortvrindt R, Smitz J, Devroey P (2001) Supernumerary pre-ovulatory follicular reduction as measure to avoid multiple pregnancy after ovulation induction. Fertil Steril 76:820–822

Armstrong DG, Webb R (1997) Ovarian follicular dominance: the role of intraovarian growth factors and novel proteins. Rev Reprod 2:139–146

Asselin E, Xiao CW, Wang YF, Tsang BK (2000) Mammalian follicular development and atresia: role of apoptosis. Biol Signals Recept 9:87–95

Baird DT (1987) A model for follicular selection and ovulation: lessons from superovulation. J Steroid Biochem 27:15–23

Barnes FL, Kausche A, Tiglias J, et al (1996) Production of embryos from in-vitro matured primary human oocytes. Fertil Steril 65:1151–1156

Barroso G, Oehninger S, Monzo A, Kolm P, Gibbons WE, Muasher SJ (2001) High FSH: LH ratio and low LH levels in basal cycle day 3: impact on follicular development and IVF outcome. J Assist Reprod Genet 18:499–505

Blondin P, Sirard MA (1995) Oocyte and follicular morphology as determining characteristics for developmental competence in bovine oocytes. Mol Reprod Dev 41:54–62

Brown JB (1978) Pituitary control of ovarian function: concepts derived from gonadotropin therapy. Aust NZ J Obstet Gynaecol 18:47–54

Cha KY, Chian RC (1998) Maturation in vitro of immature human oocytes for clinical use. Hum Reprod Update 4:103–120

Cha KY, Koo JJ, Ko JJ, Choi DH, Han SY, Yoon TK (1991) Pregnancy after in vitro fertilization of human follicular oocytes collected from nonstimulated cycles, their culture in vitro and their transfer in a donor oocyte program. Fertil Steril 55:109–113

Chian RC, Buckett WM, Tulandi T, Tan SL (2000) Prospective randomized study of human chorionic gonadotrophin priming before immature oocyte retrieval from unstimulated women with polycystic ovarian syndrome. Hum Reprod 15:165–170

Child TJ, Gulekli B, Tan SL (2001) Success during in vitro maturation (IVM) of oocyte treatment is dependent on the numbers of oocytes retrieved which are predicted by early follicular phase transvaginal ultrasound measurement of the antral follicle count and peak ovarian stromal blood flow velocity. Hum Reprod 16(Abstract Book 1):41

Cobo AC, Requena A, Neuspiller F, Aragones M, Mercader A, Navarro J, Simon C, Remohi J, Pellicer A (1999) Maturation in vitro of human oocytes from unstimulated cycles: selection of the optimal day for ovum retrieval based on follicular size. Hum Reprod 14:1864–1868

de Ziegler D, Jaaskelainen AS, Brioschi PA, Fanchin R, Bulletti C (1998) Synchronisation of endogenous and exogenous FSH stimuli in controlled ovarian hyperstimulation (COH). Hum Reprod 13:561–564

Driancourt M (1991) Follicular dynamics in sheep and cattle. Theriogenology 35:55–79

Dumesic DA, Damario MA, Session DR, Famuyide A, Lesnick TG, Thornhill AR, McNeilly AS (2001) Ovarian morphology and serum hormone markers as predictors of ovarian follicle recruitment by gonadotropins for in vitro fertilisation. J Clin Endocrinol Metab 86:2538–2543

Ethier JF, Findlay JK (2001) Roles of activin and its signal transduction mechanisms in reproductive tissues. Reprod 121:667–675

Galli C, Moor RM (1991) Gonadotrophin requirements for the in-vitro maturation of sheep oocytes and their subsequent embryonic development. Theriogenology 35:1083–1093

Gougeon A (1986) Dynamics of follicular growth in the human: a model from preliminary results. Hum Reprod 1:81–87

Gougeon A (1996) Regulation of ovarian follicular development in primates: facts and hypotheses. Endocrine Rev 17:121–155

Hildebrandt NB, Host E, Mikkelsen AL (2001) Pain experience during transvaginal aspiration of immature oocytes. Acta Obstet Gynecol Scand 80:1043–1045

Hillier SG, Tetsuka M (1997) Role of androgens in follicle maturation and atresia. Baillieres Clin Obstet Gynaecol 11:249–260

Host E, Mikkelsen AL, Lindenberg S, Smidt-Jensen S (2000) Apoptosis in human cumulus cells in relation to maturation stage and cleavage of the corresponding oocyte. Acta Obstet Gynecol Scan 79:936–940

Johnston LA, O'Brien SJ, Wildt DE (1989) In-vitro maturation and fertilization of domestic cat follicular oocytes. Gamete Res 24:343–356

Lass A, Silye R, Abrams DC, Krausz T, Hovatta O, Margara R, Winston RML (1997) Follicular density in ovarian biopsy of infertile women: a novel method to assess ovarian reserve. Hum Reprod 12:1028–1031

Lu KH, Shi DS, Jiang HS, Goulding D, Boland MP, Roche JF (1991) Comparison of the development capacity of bovine oocytes from superovulated and non-stimulated heifers. Theriogenology 35:234

Mattioli M, Bacci ML, Galeati G, Seren E (1991) Effects of LH and FSH on the maturation of pig oocytes in vitro. Theriogenology 36:95–105

McNatty KP, Smith DM, Makris A, Osathanondh R, Ryan KJ (1979) The microenvironment of the human antral follicle: interrelationships among the steroid levels in antral fluid, the population of granulosa cells, and the status of the oocyte in vivo and in vitro. J Clin Endocrinol Metab 49:851–860

Mikkelsen AL, Lindenberg S (2001) Benefit of FSH priming of women with PCOS to the in vitro maturation procedure and the outcome: a randomised prospective study. Reproduction 122:587–592

Mikkelsen AL, Smith SD, Lindenberg S (1998) In vitro maturation of immature human oocytes. Hum Reprod 13(Abstract Book 1):23–24

Mikkelsen AL, Smith SD, Lindenberg S (1999) In-vitro maturation of human oocytes from regularly menstruating women may be successful without follicle stimulating hormone priming. Hum Reprod 14:1847–1851

Mikkelsen AL, Host E, Lindenberg S (2001) Incidence of apoptosis in granulosa cells from immature human follicles. Reproduction 122:481–486

Nakahara K, Saito H, Saito T, Ito M, Ohta N, Takahashi T, Hiroi M (1997) The incidence of apoptotic bodies in membrana granulosa can predict prognosis of ova from patients participating in in vitro fertilization programs. Fertil Steril 68:312–317

Oktay K, Briggs D, Gosden RG (1997) Ontogeny of follicle-stimulating hormone receptor gene expression in isolated human ovarian follicles. J Clin Endocrinol Metab 82:3748–3751

Parrott JA, Skinner MK (1998a) Developmental and hormonal regulation of keratinocyte growth factor expression and action in the ovarian follicle. Endocrinol 139:228–235

Parrott JA, Skinner MK (1998b) Thecal cell-granulosa cell interactions involve a positive feedback loop among keratinocyte growth factor, hepatocyte growth factor, and Kit Ligand during ovarian follicular development. Endocrinol 139:2240–2245

Pavlok A, Lucas-Hahn A, Niemann H (1992) Fertilization and developmental competence of bovine oocytes derived from different categories of antral follicles. Mol Reprod Dev 31:63–67

Richards JS (2001) Perspective: the ovarian follicle – a perspective in 2001. Endocrinology 142:2184–2193

Rizk B, Smitz J (1992) Ovarian hyperstimulation syndrome after superovulation using GnRH agonists for IVF and related procedure. Hum Reprod 7:320–327

Russell JB, Knezevich KM, Fabian KF, Dickson JA (1997) Unstimulated immature oocyte retrieval: early versus midfollicular endometrial priming. Fertil Steril 67:616–620

Schats R, Schoemaker J (2001) The use of GnRH agonists. In: Gardner, Weissman A, Howles C, Shoham Z (eds) Textbook of assisted reproductive technology. Martin Dunitz, London, pp 483–491

Schipper I, Hop WC, Fauser BC (1998) The follicle-stimulating hormone (FSH) threshold/window concept examined by different interventions with exogenous FSH during the follicular phase of the normal menstrual cycle: duration, rather than magnitude, of FSH increase affects follicle development. J Clin Endocrinol Metab 83:1292–1298

Schramm RD, Bavister BD (1994) Follicle-stimulating hormone priming of rhesus monkeys enhances meiotic and developmental competence of oocytes matured in vitro. Biol Reprod 51:904–912

Scott RT, Toner JP, Muasher SJ, Oehninger S, Robinson S, Rosenwaks Z (1989) Follicle-stimulating hormone levels on cycle day 3 are predictive of in vitro fertilisation outcome. Fertil Steril 51:651–654

Seifer DB, Scott RT Jr, Bergh PA, Abrogast LK, Friedman CI, Mack CK, Danforth DR (1999) Women with declining ovarian reserve may demonstrate a decrease in day 3 serum inhibin B before a rise in day 3 follicle-stimulating hormone. Fertil Steril 72:63–65

Sirard MA, Picard L, Dery M, Coenen K, Blondin P (1999) The time interval between FSH administration and ovarian aspiration influences the development of cattle oocytes. Theriogenology 51:699–708

Smith SD, Mikkelsen AL, Lindenberg S (2000) Development of human oocytes matured in vitro for 28 or 36 hours. Fertil Steril 73:541–544

Smitz J, Nogueira D, Cortvrindt R, de Matos DG (2001) Oocyte in vitro maturation: state of the ART and basic requirements. In: Gardner, Weissman, Howles, Shoham (eds) Textbook of assisted reproductive technology. Martin Dunitz LTD, London, pp 107–137

Sokka TA, Hamalainen TM, Kaipia A, Warren DW, Huhtaniemi IT (1996) Development of luteinizing hormone action in the perinatal rat ovary. Biol Reprod 55:663–670

Trounson A, Wood C, Kausche A (1994) In vitro maturation and the fertilization and developmental competence of oocytes recovered from untreated polycystic ovarian patients. Fertil Steril 62:353–362

Trounson A, Anderiesz C, Jones G (2001) Maturation of human oocytes in vitro and their developmental competence. Reproduction 121:51–75

Wynn P, Picton HM, Krapez JA, Rutherford AJ, Balen AH, Gosden RG (1998) Pretreatment with follicle stimulating hormone promotes the numbers of human oocytes reaching metaphase II by in-vitro maturation. Hum Reprod 13:3132–3138

Younis AI, Brackett BG, Fayrer-Hosken RA (1989) Influence of serum and hormone on bovine oocyte maturation and fertilization in vitro. Gamete Res 23:189–201

Yuan W, Giudice LC (1997) Programmed cell death in human ovary is a function of follicle and corpus luteum status. J Clin Endocrinol Metab 82:3148–3155

Zeleznik AJ, Kubik CJ (1986) Ovarian responses in macaques to pulsatile infusion of follicle-stimulating hormone (FSH) and luteinizing hormone: increased sensitivity of the maturing follicle to FSH. Endocrinology 119:2025–2032

11 FF-MAS and Its Role in Mammalian Oocyte Maturation

C. Grøndahl

11.1 Introduction 177
11.2 Results and Discussion 180
11.3 Conclusion 190
References 190

11.1 Introduction

Fertilization of the mammalian oocytes completes the meiotic process that has been initiated at the time of oocyte formation in fetal life. The meiotic cell division is a prerequisite for sexual reproduction and constitutes a unique cell division not only to produce gametes but also to control the successful interaction of gametes. The pituitary hormones follicle-stimulating hormone (FSH) and luteinizing hormone (LH) are generally believed to control the overall regulation of ovarian physiology and thereby also control the processes of follicular growth, oocytes maturation, and follicle ovulation. The mechanism by which the oocytes are inhibited from resuming meiosis in the ovarian follicular environment has not been completely elucidated. The follicle fluid contains purines, e.g., hypoxanthine, that are considered to be important inhibitory substances of oocyte maturation (Downs 1993; Downs et al. 1985; Eppig et al. 1985).

Gap junctions connecting the oocyte with the surrounding cumulus cells within the follicle allow the transfer of small molecules from somatic cells to the germ cell and vice versa. The inhibitory principle has been putatively attributed to the follicular wall (Leibfried and First 1980), granulosa cells (Tsafriri and Channing 1975), and theca cells (Richard and Sirard 1996), but the nature of the inhibitory mechanism has not yet been identified.

Similarly, the mechanism by which the oocyte overcomes meiotic arrest is not well understood. Several authors have reported evidence that cumulus cells can produce a gonadotropin-dependent positive stimulus to meiotic resumption (Downs et al. 1988; Guoliang et al. 1994; Byskov et al. 1997). In 1995, it was suggested that a small group of intermediates of the cholesterol biosynthesis might represent the physiological signal, which originates in the somatic compartment of the follicle and instructs the oocyte to reinitiate the meiotic cycle. The lipophilic molecule that was found in the human follicular fluid was identified as 4,4-dimethyl-5α-cholest-8,14,24-trien-3β-ol and known as follicular fluid meiosis-activating sterol (FF-MAS) (Byskov et al. 1995).

It is well established that the second messenger cyclic adenosine monophosphate (cAMP) is involved in the signal transduction of oocyte maturation. It has been shown by many groups that cAMP is essential in the meiotic arrest and that a drop in the intracellular level of cAMP leads to the initiation of resumption of meiosis in mammalian oocytes (Eppig 1989). The spontaneous maturation in vitro can be blocked or delayed by addition of several agents, such as cAMP derivatives and phosphodiesterase (PDE) inhibitors, which modulate the intraoocyte cAMP level and subsequently meiotic resumption (Cho et al. 1974; Eppig and Downs 1984; Grøndahl et al. 2000b), or by increasing the level of cAMP by activators of the adenylate cyclase such as forskolin (Dekel et al. 1984).

Subtype 3 PDE (PDE3) and subtype 4 PDE (PDE4) are thought to be selectively expressed and regulated in the cumulus oocyte complex PDE3 being predominant expressed in the oocyte while PDE 4 is expressed mainly in the granulosa cells. Thus, it has been suggested that meiotic resumption requires high cAMP levels in the granulosa cells and low or decreasing levels in the oocyte, and that such opposing levels of cAMP may result from the selective expression and regulation of these PDEs in the two compartments of the cumulus oocyte complex (Tsafriri et al. 1996).

The resumption of meiotic maturation in oocytes involves changes in the phosphorylation status of a series of specific proteins with kinase and phosphatase activity. Among these is the cytoplasmic factor, maturation-promoting factor (MPF), known to lead to germinal vesicle (GV) breakdown (GVBD). MPF is a heterodimer of a regulatory subunit, cyclin B, and a catalytic subunit, $p34^{cdc2}$. Prophase-arrested mouse oocytes contain complexes of cyclin B and $p34^{cdc2}$ that can be activated by a dephosphorylation process, thereby probably triggering histone H1 kinase activity. This general principle is shared among all investigated vertebrates, including fish and frog oocytes (Yamashita 2000). Moreover, the kinase mos and enzymes of the mitogen-activated protein kinase (MAPK) family are involved in meiotic maturation of oocytes. MAPK, also called extracellular regulated kinase (ERK), is a serine/threonine kinase activated by the c-mos protooncogene protein kinase during mouse oocyte maturation (Verlhac et al. 1996).

It is well established that oocytes liberated from fully grown follicles for a number of species including humans are capable of undergoing spontaneous meiotic maturation in vitro; however, the subsequent embryonic development in vitro varies tremendously among species, and so far the human embryonic competence of in vitro maturation has been poor (Pincus and Enzmann 1935; Edwards 1965; Cha et al. 1991; Zhang et al. 1993; Trounson et al. 1994, 2001; Barnes et al. 1995; Weston et al. 1996; Russell et al. 1997).

It is hypothesized that FF-MAS is involved in physiological resumption of meiosis in vivo. Furthermore, it is hypothesized that the two processes spontaneous and induced maturation is vastly different and that MAS-induced maturation leads to higher oocyte quality leading to better embryos with higher developmental potential. Finally, it is hypothesized that FF-MAS may be an important contribution to the field of reproduction and have clinical applications to the treatment of human infertility.

In the following paragraphs, data obtained with FF-MAS in vitro will be reviewed and discussed.

11.2 Results and Discussion

11.2.1 Endogenous Levels of FF-MAS and Influence of FSH and LH/hCG

The formation of FF-MAS in vivo has been studied (C. Grøndahl et al. 2002, submitted). The pituitary hormones FSH and LH are generally believed to control the overall regulation of ovarian physiology and thereby also control the processes of follicular growth, oocyte maturation, and follicle ovulation. FF-MAS is known to be formed by conversion of lanosterol by the enzyme lanosterol 14-alpha-demethylase and has been found in follicular fluid in micromolar concentrations (Byskov et al. 1999). This study was undertaken to further investigate whether FF-MAS and related sterols are part of reproductive physiology and to substantiate whether FF-MAS is part of the gonadotropin signaling. The level of FF-MAS in rabbit ovarian tissue was measured in prepubertal females after different priming protocols to observe whether the level of FF-MAS was under gonadotropin regulation. The absolute amounts of FF-MAS in the ovaries were determined by chloroform-methanol extraction of the tissue, followed by normal phase HPLC fractionation of the lipid extract, and, finally, quantification by reversed phase HPLC. The level of FF-MAS in the ovary is expressed relative to the total lipid content of the ovary (ng FF-MAS per mg of total lipid extract). The basic level of FF-MAS in ovarian tissue of pre-pubertal rabbits was measured to 3.2+/–0.8 mean +/–standard error of mean (SEM) ng FF-MAS per mg total lipid extract. This basic level was not significantly elevated after FSH priming; however, after FSH stimulation followed by hCG (LH activity) the FF-MAS level in ovarian tissue was observed to rapidly and significantly increase and was constantly elevated from 1 h to 12 h after human chorionic gonadotropin (hCG) exposure (see Fig. 1).

In conclusion, LH is observed to be the key gonadotropin influencing FF-MAS activity in the ovary, providing evidence for the hypothesis that FF-MAS is part of ovarian physiology and plays a role in oocytes maturation in vivo. Moreover, it is speculated that FF-MAS has a role in vivo as a second messenger for LH with respect to resumption of oocytes meiosis. In vivo, the oocytes will resume meiosis as a consequence of the mid-cycle rise in gonadotropins (Adashi 1994). Especially

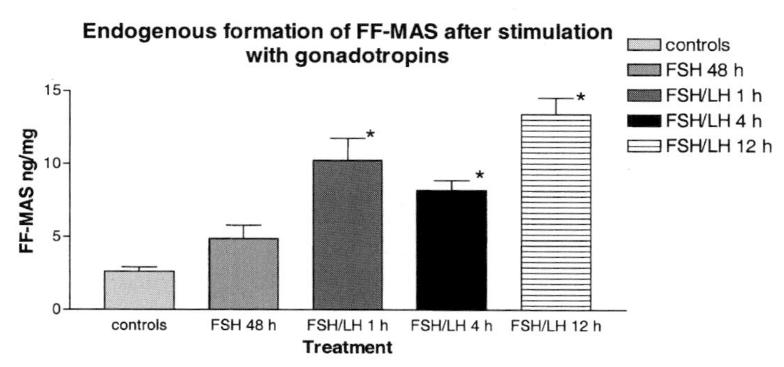

Fig. 1. The measured content of FF-MAS in ovarian tissue in pre-pubertal rabbits in non-stimulated animals, in animals after FSH stimulation, and following different time points after both FSH and hCG stimulation, 1 h, 4 h, and 12 h, respectively. Note that FSH alone has no significant influence on FF-MAS levels; however, hCG/LH preparation has a significant increase (*$p<0.01$) in the FF-MAS level and a significant rise is noted already after 1 h of hCG/LH stimulation

the LH rise/peak will trigger a timed resumption of meiosis leading to synchronous nuclear and cytoplasmic maturation visualized as nucleus membrane breakdown (GVBD) and extrusion of the first polar body, producing a fully mature metaphase-II oocyte at the time of follicle ovulation that is ready for fertilization.

11.2.2 Effect of FF-MAS on In Vitro Oocyte Maturation

The effect of FF-MAS on in vitro oocyte maturation has been investigated in meiotically arrested oocytes in mice (see Grøndahl et al. 1998 for details).

The percentage of germinal vesicle breakdown followed a clear dose-response relationship. FF-MAS in the concentrations of 0.7 and 7 μM significantly ($p<0.05$) stimulated the germinal vesicle breakdown in both naked oocytes and cumulus-enclosed oocytes, while the lowest test concentration, of 0.07 μM, was not significantly different from the controls. Figure 2 illustrates the percentage of mouse oocytes undergoing germinal vesicle breakdown after 24 h of in vitro culture with FF-MAS 0.07, 0.7, and 7 μM compared with controls of naked oocytes. Thus,

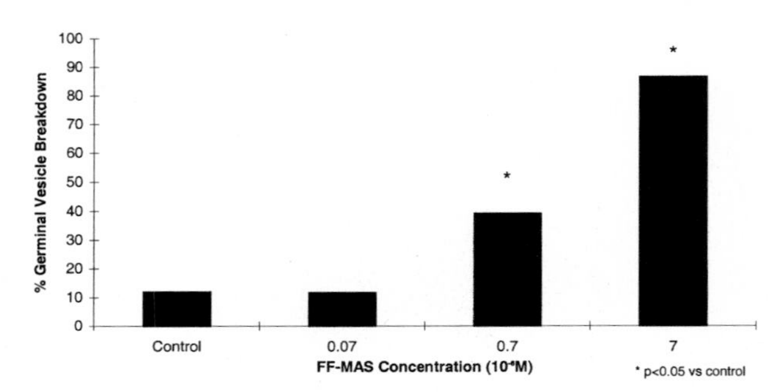

Fig. 2. FF-MAS dose-dependently induces meiosis in mouse oocytes in vitro. Culture of naked mouse oocytes in vitro for 24 h with FF-MAS in the concentration of 7 μM significantly increased the onset of germinal vesicle breakdown from 12% in the controls to 86%

synthetic FF-MAS has been observed to induce oocyte maturation in a dose-dependent manner in oocytes from mice regardless of the inhibitory agent being hypoxanthine, isobutylmethylxanthine (IBMX), or dibutryryl (db)cAMP. In a similar manner, FF-MAS has been found to signal meiotic resumption in rat oocytes (Hegele-Hartung et al. 2001) and cattle oocytes (Avery et al. 1999).

Kinetic investigation of FF-MAS effect of meiotic resumption in denuded and cumulus enclosed mouse oocytes has also been performed (C. Grøndahl et al. 2002, submitted).

The culturing of FF-MAS for a specific length of time, followed by FF-MAS wash out and subsequent culture for 22 h, revealed a marked difference in the response of denuded and cumulus-enclosed mouse oocytes (see Fig. 3a and 3b). A significant effect of FF-MAS was noted 2 h after culture in denuded oocytes, whereas no significant effect in cumulus-enclosed oocytes was noted at this point in time. After 4 h of culture, almost full effect (75% GVB) was noted in naked oocytes, in contrast to cumulus-enclosed oocytes, where only slight, although significant, activation was noted. An apparent difference in E-max for naked and cumulus enclosed oocytes at the FF-MAS concentration of 30 μM (~80% GVB vs 60% GVB, respectively) was also observed.

It has been shown that arrested cumulus-enclosed oocytes, but not naked oocytes, can be induced to resume meiosis by either treatment with FSH or epithelial growth factor (EGF) (Downs et al. 1988;

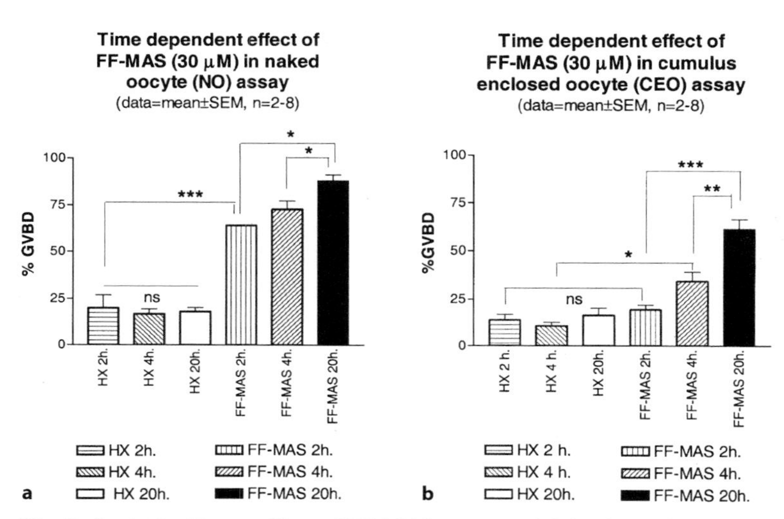

Fig. 3a,b. A significant effect of FF-MAS was noted 2 h after culture in denuded oocytes, whereas no significant effect in cumulus-enclosed oocytes was noted at this point in time. After 4 h of culture almost full effect (75% GVB) was noted in naked oocytes in contrast to cumulus-enclosed oocytes, where only slight activation, although significant, was noted. Note also the apparent difference in E-max for naked and cumulus-enclosed oocytes at the FF-MAS concentration 30 μM (~80% GVB vs 60% GVB, respectively)

Morishige et al. 1993; Singh et al. 1993; Merriman et al. 1998). In contrast, LH/hCG has little effect, if any, on the isolated cumulus–oocyte complex (Downs et al. 1988) – it requires a full functional follicle to signal, possibly because the oocytes down-regulate LH receptors in the cumulus cells adjacent to the oocyte (Eppig et al. 1997). Downs et al. (2001) also found profound differences in the effect of FF-MAS on naked and cumulus-enclosed oocytes, but did not, however, observe a significant effect on cumulus enclosed oocytes.

11.2.3 Cascade of Endogenous Occurring Meiotic Active Sterols In Vivo

The natural cascade of FF-MAS-related molecules that are meiosis-active has been studied and reported (Grøndahl et al. 2001).

FF-MAS was first identified in 1995 (Byskov et al.) as an endogenously molecule in human follicular fluid possessing the ability to induce meiosis in arrested mouse oocytes when cultured in vitro.

UV-guided fractionation of human follicular fluid resulted in isolation of four sterols, besides FF-MAS and T-MAS (sterol previously isolated from testicular tissue), in microgram amounts. Characterization of the sterols by ultraviolet (UV) nuclear magnetic resonance (NMR) and mass spectrometry (MS) identified them as closely related structurally to FF-MAS and T-MAS, i.e., either C4-methylated and/or C24-reduced derivatives. The sterols were all found to possess meiotic-inducing activity and constitute a prominent addition to the family of naturally occurring meiosis activating sterols.

The sterols are all considered intermediates on the biosynthetic pathway between lanosterol and cholesterol, and are present in micromolar concentrations in follicular fluid in the range of approximately 0.5 to 3 μM.

When hypoxanthine-arrested mouse oocytes are exposed to these sterols, they induce meiotic maturation when dosed at a concentration of 10 μM to a similar efficacy between 60% and 80% GVB in mouse oocyte in vitro assay, as previously described (Grøndahl et al. 1998).

These observations expand our knowledge about the potential signaling molecules involved in oocytes maturation. The sterol-induced oocyte maturation is potentially not exclusively brought about by a single molecule (FF-MAS) but more likely by a family of closely related MAS sterols that are intimately connected metabolically. The family members all possess the ability to induce resumption of meiosis, at least in vitro, with comparable potency. Thus, speculatively, they could signal through the same route.

11.2.4 Effect of FF-MAS on Chromosome and Spindle Organization In Vitro

Chromosome and spindle organization has been investigated in mouse oocytes cultured in vitro with FF-MAS (see Hegele-Hartung et al. 1999 for details).

In spontaneously matured oocytes, the chromosomes were all lined up as metaphase bivalents at the spindle equator in metaphase I spindles. Hardly any oocytes had chromosomes displaced from the equator. A few oocytes in late telophase were found with a typical midbody tubulin pattern. Chromosomes in the polar body or oocyte were sometimes arranged in a half-circle, which is typical for this stage and no indicator of disjunction.

In the FF-MAS-matured oocytes, anaphase and telophase oocytes possessed normal anaphase/telophase spindles in which all chromosomes had migrated to the spindle poles, and no lagging as indicator of non-disjunction was observed. Oocytes in metaphase II exhibited the typical barrel-shaped spindle with flat spindle poles, and no disturbances in chromosome alignment at the equator were noticed. Microtubular asters in metaphase II oocytes were not significantly increased compared to those in spontaneously matured control oocytes.

In conclusion, in vitro FF-MAS-induced maturation exhibits all the characteristic features of meiosis with respect to the normal appearance of the spindle apparatus and the progression to and arrest at metaphase II. High quality of oocytes was also apparent from the correct alignment of chromosomes at the spindle equator in FF-MAS-matured oocytes, since dispersal and displacement of chromosomes are often signs of predisposition to non-disjunction in response to spindle damage and aging.

11.2.5 Effect of FF-MAS on In Vitro Oocyte Fertilization

The effect of FF-MAS on in vitro oocyte fertilization has been investigated in mice (see Hegele-Hartung et al. 1998 for details).

The fertilization rate was significantly ($p<0.001$) higher in the FF-MAS 10-μM group compared to the controls. Based on the studies conducted, the overall fertilization rate (estimate±SEM) was 27.1±2.0 in the control group and 39.0±2.2 in the FF-MAS 10-μM group. The mean stimulation factor was calculated to be 1.7±0.2

Comparison between fertilization rates revealed that FF-MAS 10 μM used for in vitro maturation resulted in significantly ($p<0.001$) higher fertilization rates than in vivo-matured oocytes. Based on all the studies conducted, the mean stimulation factor was found to be 2.1±0.2.

Thus, the fertilization rate in mouse oocytes cultured in vitro with FF-MAS 10 μM was significantly higher than both in vitro spontaneously maturing oocytes and in vivo-matured oocytes.

11.2.6 Effect of FF-MAS on Human Oocyte Maturation

The effect of FF-MAS on human in vitro oocyte maturation has been investigated in immature oocytes aspirated from in vitro fertilization (IVF) patients diagnosed as polycystic ovarian syndrome (PCOS) patients (see Grøndahl et al. 2000a for details).

Following in vitro maturation of aspirated oocytes, the progression of nuclear and cytoplasmic maturation was examined by light microscopy and electron microscopy, respectively. Nuclear maturation was observed at 0, 22, 30, and 40 h after aspiration, where the oocytes were classified as germinal vesicle stage, germinal vesicle breakdown, or metaphase II stage. The number of cortical granules was considered as a morphological criterion for cytoplasmic maturation and was evaluated at 0 and 30 h.

The distribution of oocytes at various stages of nuclear maturity following 30 h of culture is shown in Fig. 4. Following in vitro maturation for 22 h, 50% of the oocytes treated with FF-MAS 20 μM, and 75% of the oocytes in the control group had resumed meiosis. However, after 30 h, 67% of the oocytes in the FF-MAS group had reached the metaphase II stage, which was significantly ($p<0.05$) higher than the 29% in the control group. In addition, 29% of the oocytes in the control group had degenerated after 30 h. At 40 h, the proportion of oocytes in the different stages was similar in the control and FF-MAS groups.

Studies are currently being undertaken to investigate the cytoplasmic maturation in human oocytes exposed to FF-MAS. In conclusion, FF-MAS exposed to human oocytes from PCOS patients for 30 h had the observed effect that the frequency of fully matured metaphase II oocytes was found to be significantly higher among oocytes cultured in vitro

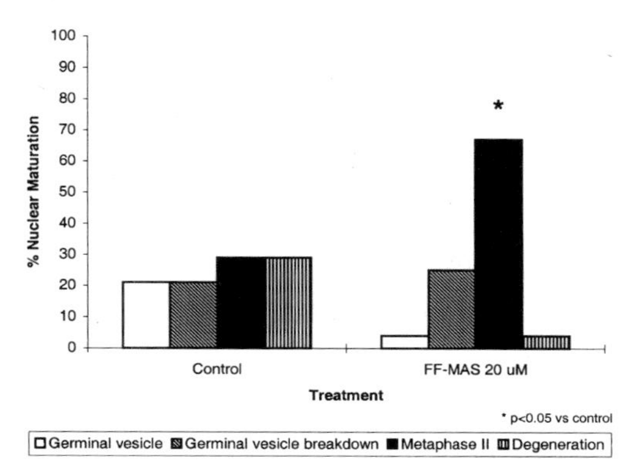

Fig. 4. The progression of nuclear maturation after 30 h culture of immature human oocytes aspirated from 8- to -12-mm follicles in patients diagnosed as PCOS. Note that after 30 h, the frequency of fully matured metaphase II oocytes was found to be significantly higher among oocytes cultured in vitro with FF-MAS 20 μM than among the spontaneously matured oocytes. In addition, FF-MAS-mediated matured oocytes displayed less degeneration

with FF-MAS 20 μM than among the spontaneously matured oocytes. Larger studies of oocytes from normal women cultured in vitro are needed to further explore the effect of FF-MAS in human oocytes.

11.2.7 MAS Signaling Pathways

The signaling pathway of spontaneous and MAS-induced resumption of meiosis has been investigated in mouse oocytes (see Grøndahl et al. 2000b and Færge et al. 2001 for details).

The purpose of this study was to examine the hypothesis that differential signal transduction mechanisms exist for FF-MAS induced and spontaneous in vitro resumption of meiosis in mouse oocytes. Mouse oocytes were dissected from ovaries originating from mice primed with FSH 48 h prior to oocyte collection. Mechanically denuded GV oocytes were in vitro matured in medium supplemented with hypoxanthine and FF-MAS or allowed to mature spontaneously: both groups were exposed to individual compounds known to inhibit specific targets in the cell. After 20–22 h in vitro maturation, the resumption of meiosis was

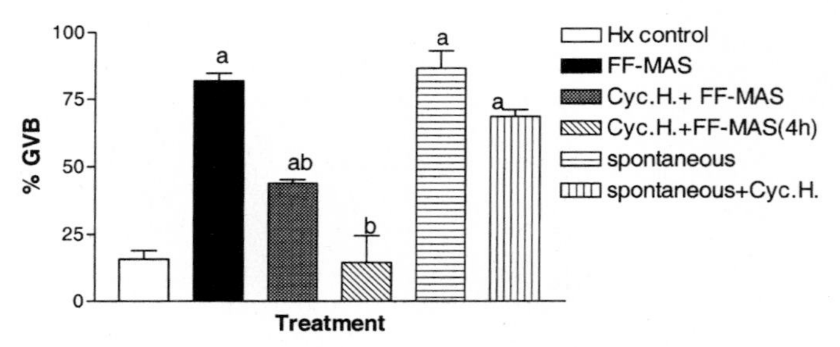

Fig. 5. The effect of cycloheximide treatment simultaneously with or 4 h before FF-MAS-mediated oocyte maturation on naked oocytes cultured in vitro. Number of oocytes: n=245, 139, 142, 262, 125 and 139 for Hx controls; FF-MAS-positive controls, 4 h; cycloheximide+FF-MAS, 0 h; cycloheximide+FF-MAS, 4 h; spontaneous; and spontaneous+cycloheximide, respectively. *Bars* and *error bars* represent mean %GVB±SD of three consecutive trials. *a* indicates that treatment group is significant different to Hx controls and *b* indicates that treatment group is significant different to FF-MAS treated positive controls assessed by ANOVA followed by pair-wise comparison using Student's *t*-test. Note that the FF-MAS (10 μM)-mediated resumption of meiosis is significantly influenced by cycloheximide (50 μg/ml) at simultaneous administration of cycloheximide and FF-MAS and completely blocked by 4 h pretreatment with cycloheximide (4 h), in contrast to spontaneous maturation that is unaffected by cycloheximide. *CycH*, cycloheximide

assessed as the frequency of oocytes in GVBD stage. MAS-induced maturation was completely blocked by protein synthesis inhibition (see Fig. 5), whereas transcription of DNA to RNA was not observed to be involved in MAS signaling. Cholera toxin was observed to inhibit MAS-induced, but not spontaneous maturation (see Fig. 6), suggesting a putative G-protein-coupled receptor mechanism of FF-MAS. Pertussis toxin did not influence resumption of meiosis in either of the two groups. Dibutyryl cyclic GMP (dbcGMP) inhibited FF-MAS-induced GVBD, but not spontaneous GVBD, whereas the subtype 5 phosphodiesterase (PDE5) inhibitor zaprinast inhibited GVBD in both groups. Addition of the mitogen-activated protein kinase (MAPK) inhibitor inhibited FF-MAS induced GVBD, but not spontaneous GVBD. Both MAPKs, ERK1 and ERK2, were phosphorylated under FF-MAS-induced meiotic resumption in contrast to spontaneous meiotic resumption, where ERK1 and ERK2 phosphorylation occurred 2 h after GVBD

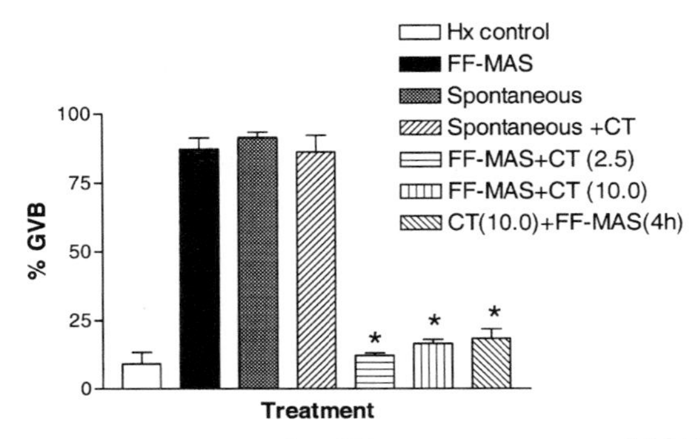

Fig. 6. The effect of cholera toxin (CT) on spontaneous and MAS-mediated oocyte maturation in naked oocytes cultured in vitro in either Hx-free medium (spontaneous) or Hx-medium (FF-MAS). Number of oocytes: n=118, 100, 119, 124, 97, 105, and 115 for spontaneous; spontaneous+CT 2.5 µg/ml; FF-MAS-positive control; Hx control; FF-MAS+CT 2.5 µg/ml, 0 h; FF-MAS+CT 10.0 µg/ml, 0 h; and CT 10.0 µg/ml+FF-MAS, 4 h, respectively. *Bars* and *error bars* represent mean±SD% GVB of three consecutive trials. Notice that by using the chi-square test, significant effects (*asterisks*) of all the various CT treatment was observed in the FF-MAS-mediated oocyte maturation, in contrast to no significant effect of CT on spontaneous maturation

(Færge et al. 2001). In conclusion, it was observed that FF-MAS depends on an active protein synthesis, acts through a cholera toxin-sensitive pathway suggestive of G-protein receptor involvement. Furthermore, it was observed that FF-MAS acts through a MAPK dependent pathway, suggesting that src-like kinase, $p21^{ras}$ and phosphoinositide signaling lie upstream of MAPK in the FF-MAS-activated signaling pathway. It is clear that striking pathway differences are present between spontaneous versus FF-MAS-induced meiotic resumption. Other groups have similarly found that induced meiotic maturation makes use of a different signaling pathway than that of spontaneous maturation (Coticchio and Flemming 1998; Leonardsen et al. 2000).

11.3 Conclusion

In summary, LH was clearly observed to be the key gonadotropin influencing FF-MAS activity in the ovary, providing evidence for the hypothesis that FF-MAS is part of ovarian physiology and plays a role in oocyte maturation in vivo. These findings support the hypothesis that two counteracting mechanisms exists in vivo: an inhibitory stimulus constantly preventing the oocytes from resuming meiosis and an activating stimulus downstream from the gonadotropic surge, especially LH, that is capable of overriding the inhibitory mechanism in vivo as the follicle approaches ovulation. A further consequence of this hypothesis is that the spontaneous maturation in vitro is far from physiology, which also is reflected in the poor developmental capabilities that in vitro-derived embryos, at least in humans, have been observed to possess up to now.

Especially cytoplasmic maturation seems to be improved by FF-MAS interaction, as seen in the enhanced fertilization rate in MAS-induced mature oocytes.

Further studies are needed to establish whether FF-MAS-induced maturation qualitatively improves oocyte maturation leading to embryos with improved embryonic competence by inducing a signaling pathway of meiotic resumption that is closer to the in vivo maturational process.

Acknowledgments. The author has reviewed scientific work made in close collaboration with and by Prof. Dr. Christa Hegele-Hartung, Drs. T. Blume, M. Lessl, Schering AG, and Drs. Inger Færge, Jan Ottesen, Anthony Murray, Philip Wahl, Jens Breinholt, Thomas Høst Hansen, Novo Nordisk A/S. Elene J Carlsen, Tina Olesen, and Anne Mette Jacobsen are thanked for skillful technical assistance.

References

Adashi EY (1994) Endocrinology of the ovary. Hum Reprod 9:815–827

Avery B, Faerge I, Grøndahl C, et al (1999) Nuclear maturation and embryo development of bovine oocytes matured in semi-defined medium supplemented with meiosis-activating sterol (MAS) (abstract). Theriogenology 51:367

Barnes FL, Crombie A, Gardner DK, et al (1995) Blastocyst development and birth after in-vitro maturation of human primary oocytes, intracytoplasmic sperm injection and assisted hatching. Hum Reprod 10:3243–3247

Byskov AG, Andersen CY, Nordholm L, et al (1995) Chemical-structure of sterols that activate oocyte meiosis. Nature 374:559–562

Byskov AG, Andersen CY, Hossaini A, et al (1997) Cumulus cells of oocyte-cumulus complexes secrete a meiosis-activating substance when stimulated with FSH. Mol Reprod Dev 46:296–305

Byskov AG, Andersen CY, Leonardsen L, et al (1999) Meiosis activating sterols (MAS) and fertility in mammals and man. J Exp Zool 285:237–242

Cha KY, Koo JJ, Ko JJ, et al (1991) Pregnancy after in vitro fertilization of human follicular oocytes collected from nonstimulated cycles, their culture in vitro and their transfer in a donor oocyte program. Fertil Steril 55:109–113

Cho WK, Stern S, Biggers JD (1974) Inhibitory effect of dibutyric cAMP on mouse oocyte maturation in vitro. J Exp Zool 187:383–386

Coticchio G, Fleming S (1998) Inhibition of phosphoinositide metabolism or chelation of intracellular calcium blocks FSH-induced but not spontaneous meiotic resumption in mouse oocytes. Dev Biol 203:201–209

Dekel N, Aberdam E, Sherizly I (1984) Spontaneous maturation in vitro of cumulus-enclosed rat oocytes is inhibited by forskolin. Biol Reprod 31:244–250

Downs SM (1993) Purine control of mouse oocyte maturation – evidence that nonmetabolized hypoxanthine maintains meiotic arrest. Mol Reprod Dev 35:82–94

Downs SM, Coleman DL, Ward-Bailey PF, et al (1985) Hypoxanthine is the principal inhibitor of murine oocyte maturation in a low molecular weight fraction of porcine follicular fluid. Proc Natl Acad Sci USA 82:454–458

Downs SM, Daniel SAJ, Bornslaegger EA, et al (1988) Induction of maturation in cumulus cell-enclosed mouse oocytes by follicle-stimulating hormone and epidermal growth factor: evidence for a positive stimulus of somatic cell origin. J Exp Zool 245:86–96

Downs SM, Ruan B, Schroepfer GJ Jr (2001) Meiosis-activating sterol and the maturation of isolated mouse oocytes. Biol Reprod 64:80–89

Edwards RG (1965) Maturation in vitro of mouse, sheep, cow, pig, rhesus monkey and human ovarian oocytes. Nature 208:349–351

Eppig JJ (1989) The participation of cyclic adenosine monophosphate (cAMP) in the regulation of meiotic maturation of oocytes in the laboratory mouse. J Reprod Fertil 38:3–8

Eppig JJ, Downs SM (1984) Chemical signals that regulate mammalian oocyte maturation. Biol Reprod 30:1–11

Eppig JJ, Ward-Bailey PF, Coleman DL (1985) Hypoxanthine and adenosine in murine ovarian follicular fluid: concentrations and activity in maintaining oocyte meiotic arrest. Biol Reprod 33:1041–1049

Eppig JJ, Wigglesworth K, Pendola F, et al (1997) Murine oocytes suppress expression of luteinizing hormone receptor messenger ribonucleic acid by granulosa cells. Biol Reprod 56:976–984

Færge I, Terry B, Kalous J, et al (2001) The resumption of meiosis induced by meiosis-activating sterol (MAS) has different signal transduction pathway than spontaneous resumption of meiosis in denuded mouse oocytes cultured in vitro. Biol Reprod 65:1751–1758

Grøndahl C, Ottesen JL, Lessl M, et al (1998) Meiosis-activating sterol promotes resumption of meiosis in mouse oocytes cultured in vitro in contrast to related oxysterols. Biol Reprod 58:1297–1302

Grøndahl C, Hansen TH, Marky-Nielsen K, et al (2000a) Human oocyte maturation in vitro is stimulated by meiosis-activating sterol. Hum Reprod 15[Suppl 5]:3–10

Grøndahl C, Lessl M, Færge I, et al (2000b) Meiosis activating sterol mediated resumption of meiosis in mouse oocytes in vitro is influenced by protein synthesis inhibition and cholera toxin. Biol Reprod 62:775–780

Grøndahl C, Breinholt J, Høst Hansen T, et al (2001) Cascade of closely related endogenous MAS sterols in human follicular fluid that possess meiotic inducing activity in mouse oocytes cultured in vitro (abstract). Fertil Steril 76(3S):457

Guoliang X, Byskov AG, Andersen CY (1994) Cumulus cells secrete a meiosis-inducing substance by stimulation with forskolin and dibutyric cyclic adenosine-monophosphate. Mol Reprod Dev 39:17–24

Hegele-Hartung C, Lessl M, Ottesen JL, et al (1998) Oocyte maturation can be induced by a synthetic meiosis activating sterol (MAS) leading to an improvement of IVF rate in mice (abstract). Hum Reprod 11:193

Hegele-Hartung C, Kuhnke J, Lessl M, et al (1999) Nuclear and cytoplasmic maturation of mouse oocytes after treatment with synthetic meiosis-activating sterol in vitro. Biol Reprod 61:1362–1372

Hegele-Hartung C, Grützner M, Lessl M, et al (2001) Activation of meiotic maturation in rat oocytes after treatment with follicular fluid meiosis-activating sterol in vitro and ex vivo. Biol Reprod 64:418–424

Leibfried L, First NL (1980) Effect of bovine and porcine follicular fluid and granulosa cells on maturation of oocytes in vitro. Biol Reprod 23:699–704

Leonardsen L, Wiersma A, Baltsen M, et al (2000) Regulation of spontaneous and induced resumption of meiosis in mouse oocytes by different intracellular pathways. J Reprod Fertil 120:377–383

Merriman JA, Whittingham DG, Carroll J (1998) The effect of follicle stimulating hormone and epidermal growth factor on the developmental capacity of in-vitro matured mouse oocytes. Hum Reprod 13:690–695

Morishige K, Kurachi H, Amemiya K, et al (1993) Menstrual stage-specific expression of epidermal growth factor and transforming growth factor-alpha in human oviduct epithelium and their role in early embryogenesis. Endocrinology 133:199–207

Pincus G, Enzmann EV (1935) The comparative behavior of mammalian eggs in vivo and in vitro. I. The activation of ovarian eggs. J Exp Med 62:655–675

Richard FJ, Sirard MA (1996) Effects of follicular cells on oocyte maturation. II. Theca cell inhibition of bovine oocyte maturation in vitro. Biol Reprod 54:22–28

Russell JB, Knezevich KM, Fabian FF, et al (1997) Unstimulated immature oocyte retrieval: early versus midfollicular endometrial priming. Fertil Steril 67:616–620

Singh B, Barbe GJ, Armstrong DT (1993) Factors influencing resumption of meiotic maturation and cumulus expansion of porcine oocyte-cumulus cell complexes in vitro. Mol Reprod Dev 36:113–119

Trounson AO, Wood C, Kausche A (1994) In vitro maturation and the fertilization and developmental competence of oocytes recovered from untreated polycystic ovarian patients. Fertil Steril 62:353–362

Trounson AO, Anderiesz C, Jones G (2001) Maturation of human oocytes in vitro and their developmental competence. Reproduction 121:51–75

Tsafriri A, Channing CP (1975) An inhibitory influence of granulosa cells and follicular fluid upon porcine oocyte meiosis in vitro. Endocrinology 96:922–927

Tsafriri A, Chun SY, Zhang R, et al (1996) Oocyte maturation involves compartmentalization and opposing changes of cAMP levels in follicular somatic and germ cells: studies using selective phosphodiesterase inhibitors. Develop Biol 178:393–402

Verlhac MH, Kubiak JZ, Weber M, et al (1996) Mos is required for MAP kinase activation and is involved in microtubule organization during meiotic maturation in the mouse. Development 122:815–822

Weston AM, Zelinski-Wooten MB, Hutchison JS, et al (1996) Developmental potential of embryos produced by in-vitro fertilization from gonadotropin-releasing hormone antagonist- treated macaques stimulated with recombinant human follicle stimulating hormone alone or in combination with luteinizing hormone. Hum Reprod 11:608–613

Yamashita M (2000) Toward modelling of a general mechanism of MPF formation during oocyte maturation in Vertebrates. Zool Sci 7:41–851

Zhang X, Zerafa A, Wong J, et al (1993) Human menopausal gonadotropin during in vitro maturation of human oocytes retrieved from small follicles enhances in vitro fertilization and cleavage rates. Fertil Steril 59:850–853

Subject Index

actin filaments 103
ADAMTS-1 50
Addison's disease 145, 147
aneuploidy 117, 122
Apaf-1 25
apoptosis 23
assisted reproduction 162, 171

Bcl-2 24
BMP-15 70

caspase family 24
caspase-9 25
caspases 25
cathepsin L 50
cell death 23
chemotherapy 138, 140
childhood cancer 138, 139
chorioallantoic membrane 15
clinical work-up 146
COX-2 46
cumulus cells 45
cyclin D2 49
cytochrome *c* 25
cytoplasmic maturation 181, 186, 190

diabetes mellitus 147

embryos 163
EP2 46

FF-MAS 177, 178, 179, 180, 181
FGF 30
follicular development 23
folliculogenesis 1, 63
Frizzled-1 54
Frizzled-4 54

gap junction 102
GDF-9 29, 47, 68, 70
genetic 142
GnRH agonist 140, 148
granulosa cells 45

HAS-2 46

IαI 47
IGF-I 31
IGFBP-3 31
in vitro maturation 163, 171
  patient selection 164
incidence 141
intermediate filaments 104
internucleosomal DNA fragmentation 25

keratinocyte growth factor (KGF) 30

MAS 87
MATER 73
microtubules 105

MIS 31
MOS 72
MPF 82

nuclear maturation 186

oocyte donation 138, 146, 150
oocyte in vitro maturation 163
oocyte-specific genes 64
oocytes 101, 111, 118, 162, 171, 177, 186
ovarian follicles 101
ovarian stimulation 163
ovulation 43

phosphatidylserine 27
PR antagonists 34
preantral follicles 3
premature ovarian failure (POF) 138, 141, 146
- causes 142
- risk 141
- treatment options 148

primary amenorrhea 139, 141
primitive germ cells 2
primordial follicles 3
- activation 11
- development 66

progesterone receptor 49
programmed cell death 23

radiotherapy 139

SR-BI (scavenger receptor class B type I) 27
surrogate motherhood 139, 148, 152

transzonal projections 102
TSG-6 46

Wnt-4 54

zona pellucida 66

Ernst Schering Research Foundation Workshop

Editors: Günter Stock
Monika Lessl

Vol. 1 *(1991)*: Bioscience⇆Society – Workshop Report
Editors: D. J. Roy, B. E. Wynne, R. W. Old

Vol. 2 (1991): Round Table Discussion on Bioscience⇆Society
Editor: J. J. Cherfas

Vol. 3 (1991): Excitatory Amino Acids and Second Messenger Systems
Editors: V. I. Teichberg, L. Turski

Vol. 4 (1992): Spermatogenesis – Fertilization – Contraception
Editors: E. Nieschlag, U.-F. Habenicht

Vol. 5 (1992): Sex Steroids and the Cardiovascular System
Editors: P. Ramwell, G. Rubanyi, E. Schillinger

Vol. 6 (1993): Transgenic Animals as Model Systems for Human Diseases
Editors: E. F. Wagner, F. Theuring

Vol. 7 (1993): Basic Mechanisms Controlling Term and Preterm Birth
Editors: K. Chwalisz, R. E. Garfield

Vol. 8 (1994): Health Care 2010
Editors: C. Bezold, K. Knabner

Vol. 9 (1994): Sex Steroids and Bone
Editors: R. Ziegler, J. Pfeilschifter, M. Bräutigam

Vol. 10 (1994): Nongenotoxic Carcinogenesis
Editors: A. Cockburn, L. Smith

Vol. 11 (1994): Cell Culture in Pharmaceutical Research
Editors: N. E. Fusenig, H. Graf

Vol. 12 (1994): Interactions Between Adjuvants, Agrochemical and Target Organisms
Editors: P. J. Holloway, R. T. Rees, D. Stock

Vol. 13 (1994): Assessment of the Use of Single Cytochrome P450 Enzymes in Drug Research
Editors: M. R. Waterman, M. Hildebrand

Vol. 14 (1995): Apoptosis in Hormone-Dependent Cancers
Editors: M. Tenniswood, H. Michna

Vol. 15 (1995): Computer Aided Drug Design in Industrial Research
Editors: E. C. Herrmann, R. Franke

Vol. 16 (1995): Organ-Selective Actions of Steroid Hormones
Editors: D. T. Baird, G. Schütz, R. Krattenmacher

Vol. 17 (1996): Alzheimer's Disease
Editors: J.D. Turner, K. Beyreuther, F. Theuring

Vol. 18 (1997): The Endometrium as a Target for Contraception
Editors: H.M. Beier, M.J.K. Harper, K. Chwalisz

Vol. 19 (1997): EGF Receptor in Tumor Growth and Progression
Editors: R. B. Lichtner, R. N. Harkins

Vol. 20 (1997): Cellular Therapy
Editors: H. Wekerle, H. Graf, J.D. Turner

Vol. 21 (1997): Nitric Oxide, Cytochromes P 450,
and Sexual Steroid Hormones
Editors: J.R. Lancaster, J.F. Parkinson

Vol. 22 (1997): Impact of Molecular Biology
and New Technical Developments in Diagnostic Imaging
Editors: W. Semmler, M. Schwaiger

Vol. 23 (1998): Excitatory Amino Acids
Editors: P.H. Seeburg, I. Bresink, L. Turski

Vol. 24 (1998): Molecular Basis of Sex Hormone Receptor Function
Editors: H. Gronemeyer, U. Fuhrmann, K. Parczyk

Vol. 25 (1998): Novel Approaches to Treatment of Osteoporosis
Editors: R.G.G. Russell, T.M. Skerry, U. Kollenkirchen

Vol. 26 (1998): Recent Trends in Molecular Recognition
Editors: F. Diederich, H. Künzer

Vol. 27 (1998): Gene Therapy
Editors: R.E. Sobol, K.J. Scanlon, E. Nestaas, T. Strohmeyer

Vol. 28 (1999): Therapeutic Angiogenesis
Editors: J.A. Dormandy, W.P. Dole, G.M. Rubanyi

Vol. 29 (2000): Of Fish, Fly, Worm and Man
Editors: C. Nüsslein-Volhard, J. Krätzschmar

Vol. 30 (2000): Therapeutic Vaccination Therapy
Editors: P. Walden, W. Sterry, H. Hennekes

Vol. 31 (2000): Advances in Eicosanoid Research
Editors: C.N. Serhan, H.D. Perez

Vol. 32 (2000): The Role of Natural Products in Drug Discovery
Editors: J. Mulzer, R. Bohlmann

Vol. 33 (2001): Stem Cells from Cord Blood, In Utero Stem Cell Development, and Transplantation-Inclusive Gene Therapy
Editors: W. Holzgreve, M. Lessl

Vol. 34 (2001): Data Mining in Structural Biology
Editors: I. Schlichting, U. Egner

Vol. 35 (2002): Stem Cell Transplantation and Tissue Engineering
Editors: A. Haverich, H. Graf

Vol. 36 (2002): The Human Genome
Editors: A. Rosenthal, L. Vakalopoulou

Vol. 37 (2002): Pharmacokinetic Challenges in Drug Discovery
Editors: O. Pelkonen, A. Baumann, A. Reichel

Vol. 38 (2002): Bioinformatics and Genome Analysis
Editors: H.-W. Mewes, B. Weiss, H. Seidel

Vol. 39 (2002): Neuroinflammation – From Bench to Bedside
Editors: H. Kettenmann, G. A. Burton, U. Moenning

Vol. 40 (2002): Recent Advances in Glucocorticoid Receptor Action
Editors: A. Cato, H. Schaecke, K. Asadullah

Vol. 41 (2002): The Future of the Oocyte: Basic and Clinical Aspects
Editors: J. Eppig, C. Hegele-Hartung, M. Lessl

Supplement 1 (1994): Molecular and Cellular Endocrinology of the Testis
Editors: G. Verhoeven, U.-F. Habenicht

Supplement 2 (1997): Signal Transduction in Testicular Cells
Editors: V. Hansson, F. O. Levy, K. Taskén

Supplement 3 (1998): Testicular Function:
From Gene Expression to Genetic Manipulation
Editors: M. Stefanini, C. Boitani, M. Galdieri, R. Geremia, F. Palombi

Supplement 4 (2000): Hormone Replacement Therapy
and Osteoporosis
Editors: J. Kato, H. Minaguchi, Y. Nishino

Supplement 5 (1999): Interferon:
The Dawn of Recombinant Protein Drugs
Editors: J. Lindenmann, W.D. Schleuning

Supplement 6 (2000): Testis, Epididymis and Technologies
in the Year 2000
Editors: B. Jégou, C. Pineau, J. Saez

Supplement 7 (2001): New Concepts in Pathology and Treatment
of Autoimmune Disorders
Editors: P. Pozzilli, C. Pozzilli, J.-F. Kapp

Supplement 8 (2001): New Pharmacological Approaches
to Reproductive Health and Healthy Ageing
Editors: W.-K. Raff, M. F. Fathalla, F. Saad

Supplement 9 (2002): Testicular Tangrams
Editors: F.F.G. Rommerts, K.J. Teerds

Supplement 10 (2002): Die Architektur des Lebens
Editors: G. Stock, M. Lessl

This series will be available on request from
Ernst Schering Research Foundation, 13342 Berlin, Germany

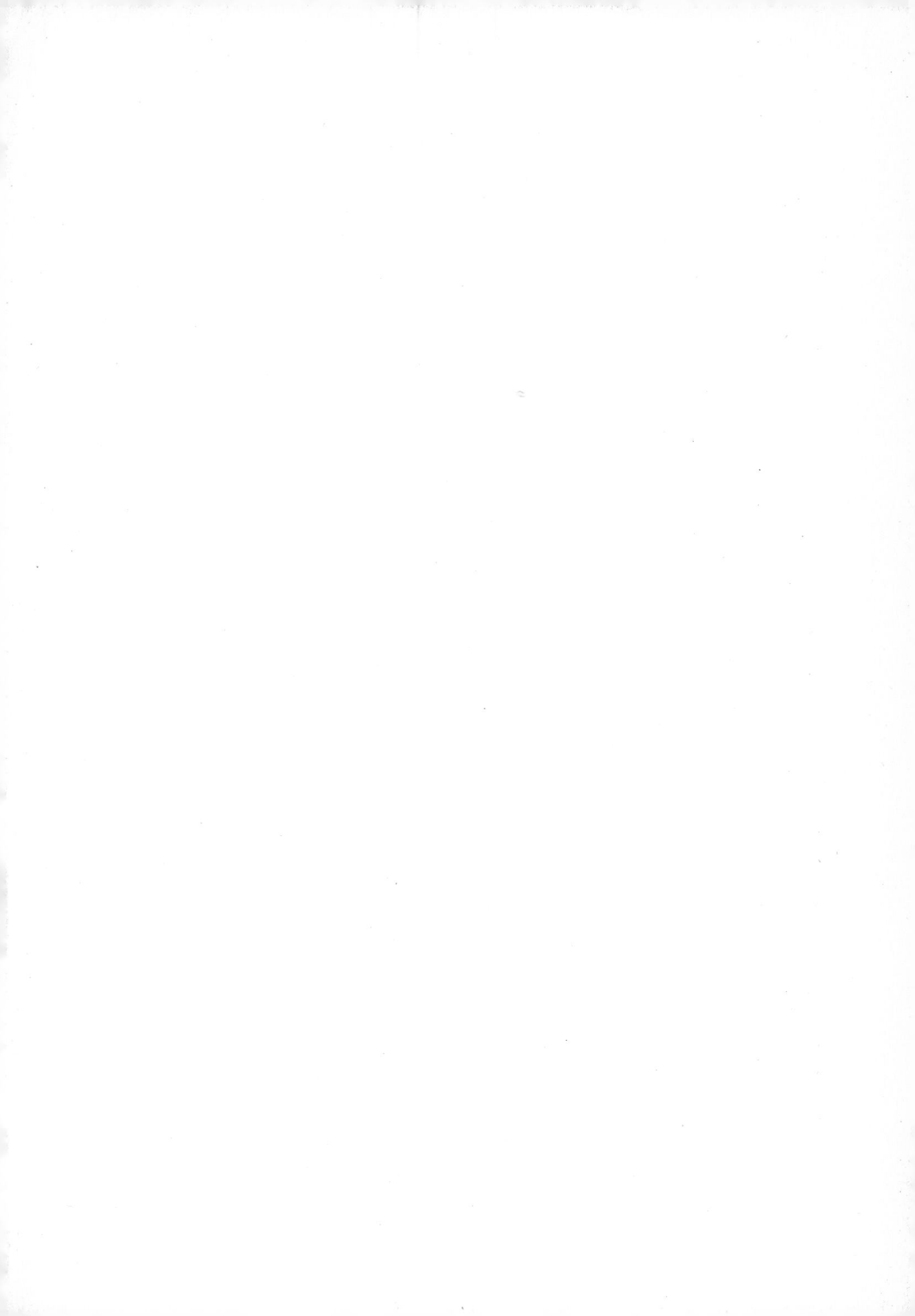